Practical Feeding of

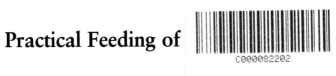

Other horse books from Blackwell Science

The Equine Athlete
How To Develop Your Horse's
Athletic Potential
Jo Hodges and Sarah Pilliner
0 632 03506 4

Getting Horses Fit
A Guide to Improving
Performance
Second Edition
Sarah Pilliner
0 632 03476 9

Horse and Stable Management
(Incorporating *Horse Care*)
Omnibus (Third) Edition
Jeremy Houghton Brown,
Vincent Powell-Smith and
Sarah Pilliner
0 632 04152 8

Equine Injury, Therapy and
Rehabilitation
Second Edition
Mary Bromiley
0 632 03608 7

Veterinary Manual for the
Performance Horse
N.S. Loving with A.M. Johnson
0 632 04166 8

Keeping Horses
The Working Owner's Guide to
Saving Time and Money
Second Edition
Susan McBane
0 632 03443 2

Coaching the Rider
Jane Houghton-Brown
0 632 03931 0

Breeding the Competition Horse
Second Edition
John Rose and Sarah Pilliner
0 632 03727 X

Natural Methods for Equine
Health
Mary Bromiley
0 632 03818 7

Equine Science, Health and
Performance
Sarah Pilliner and Zoe Davies
0 632 03913 2

Horse Business Management
Second Edition
Jeremy Houghton Brown and
Vincent Powell-Smith
0 632 03821 7

Practical Feeding
of Horses and Ponies

Sarah Pilliner
MSc, BHSI (SM)

b

**Blackwell
Science**

© 1998 Sarah Pilliner

Blackwell Science Ltd
Editorial Offices:
Osney Mead, Oxford OX2 0EL
25 John Street, London WC1N 2BL
23 Ainslie Place, Edinburgh EH3 6AJ
350 Main Street, Malden
  MA 02148 5018, USA
54 University Street, Carlton
  Victoria 3053, Australia

Other Editorial Offices:

Blackwell Wissenschafts-Verlag GmbH
Kurfürstendamm 57
10707 Berlin, Germany

Blackwell Science KK
MG Kodenmacho Building
7–10 Kodenmacho Nihombashi
Chuo-ku, Tokyo 104, Japan

First published 1998

Set in 10.5/13.5 pt Sabon
by DP Photosetting, Aylesbury, Bucks
Printed and bound in Great Britain by
MPG Books Limited, Bodmin, Cornwall

The Blackwell Science logo is a trade mark of
Blackwell Science Ltd, registered at the
United Kingdom Trade Marks Registry

DISTRIBUTORS

Marston Book Services Ltd
PO Box 269
Abingdon
Oxon OX14 4YN
(*Orders:* Tel: 01235 465500
        Fax: 01235 465555)

USA
Blackwell Science, Inc.
Commerce Place
350 Main Street
Malden, MA 02148 5018
(*Orders:* Tel: 800 759 6102
                617 388 8250
        Fax: 617 388 8255)

Canada
Copp Clark Professional
200 Adelaide Street West, 3rd Floor
Toronto, Ontario M5H 1W7
(*Orders:* Tel: 416 597 1616
                800 815 9417
        Fax: 416 597 1617)

Australia
Blackwell Science Pty Ltd
54 University Street
Carlton, Victoria 3053
(*Orders:* Tel: 03 9347 0300
        Fax: 03 9347 5001)

A catalogue record for this title
is available from the British Library

ISBN 0-632-04828-X

Library of Congress
Cataloging-in-Publication Data

Pilliner, Sarah.
  Practical feeding of horses and ponies/
Sarah Pilliner.
        p.   cm.
    Includes index.
    ISBN 0-632-04828-X
    1. Horses – Feeding and feeds.
    2. Ponies – Feeding and feeds.
    I. Title.
    SF285.5.P55   1997
    636.1′085 – dc21   97-27543
                                        CIP

Contents

Preface

Most of us want our horses to perform to the best of their ability and know that correct feeding will lead to good health and better performance. Turn the pages of any horse magazine and you are bombarded with adverts for feeds and supplements – all of which claim to be the one for your horse. We all want to do the best for our horses and people become concerned – 'Am I feeding my horse correctly?', 'Should I change my feeding regime?' Frequently, the answer to these queries lies in the practical day-to-day feeding of horses. The closer we can stick to the way Nature intended the horse to be fed, the happier and healthier the horse is likely to be.

There seem to be a multitude of problems associated with feeding horses and ponies. Some people are worried that their horse is too fat while others want their horse to carry more condition. Many owners have horses with temperament problems and hope that changing the feeding can result in a quieter, less unpredictable horse. Very often, all that is needed to put people's minds at rest and to help their horses are some simple, practical guidelines, which take the mystique out of feeding horses. *Practical Feeding of Horses and Ponies* aims to help the horse owner through this maze and to give practical advice on how to feed and get the best from your horse.

This book sets out some tips and guidelines using a blend of the art and science of feeding horses with a common-sense approach. Ultimately, it is up to you, the owner, to make the subtle adjustments to suit your own horse's individual tastes and requirements.

Part 1
Theory Versus Practice

Chapter 1
The Horse in its Natural State

The horse has evolved over millions of years to become a fleet-footed herbivore. It is an animal designed to live in herds, roaming freely over wide areas, surviving on a diet of grass, shrubs and herbs and by out-pacing its predators, much as zebras do today. This life style is reflected in the organisation of the horse's digestive system and its natural behaviour patterns. It also explains why the horse falls prey to many of the ailments associated with feeding and digestion. An understanding of its eating patterns, selective and social feeding habits and digestive function is essential if the horse is to be kept healthy and happy.

Digestive development

During the process of evolution the ancestors of the horse, cow and sheep chose a high fibre diet consisting of the leaves and stems of plants. This fibrous material contains cellulose, a complex substance which cannot be broken down by the enzymes of the digestive system. This meant that the herbivores had to develop an alternative way to release the nutrition locked up in grass. The first thing was to form a relationship with micro-organisms capable of breaking down cellulose and then to give these organisms a place to work on the cellulose (see Chapter 2). Parts of the horse's digestive tract, the caecum and colon, evolved to be larger over time to provide the organisms with a place to break down or ferment the cellulose. Horses became *hind-gut diges-ters*. However, the cow and sheep followed a different route; the stomach of these ruminant animals became enlarged, making them *fore-gut fermenters*.

Although it takes place in a different part of the gut, the process of fermentation appears to be the same in both horses and ruminants. However, horses are less efficient at digesting cellulose-rich vegetation, which is partly because the digestive tract of the cow is comparatively much bigger than that of the horse. The cow's digestive tract and its contents make up about 40% of its bodyweight, while that of the horse is only about 15% of bodyweight.

The position of the fermentation site affects the way in which the horse can utilise feed resources. For example, in the cow, the small intestine absorbs the products of fermentation. However, the horse does not have an absorption area after the fermentation site, leading to the loss of nutrients in the dung. On the plus side the horse is able to digest fat, sugar and starch efficiently in the small intestine, while the cow ferments these valuable nutrients which destroys their nutritional value.

The next step was for the horse to develop a way of gathering and processing fibrous foods before swallowing. The long, elegant head of the horse is not designed for beauty but to house its large teeth which have the job of grinding grass to a pulp. Grass and leaves contain silica, a very hard, sand-like substance. A diet of grass would quickly wear the horse's teeth down but for a substance called cement, which forms a layer resembling bone over the dentine of the tooth. This extra dental element allows the horse to munch through substantial branches with impunity. The horse also has high crowned teeth which grow continuously throughout its life to compensate for wear. The gradual changes in the shape of the horse's skull during its evolution have allowed the horse to exert substantial crushing forces and a side-to-side shearing action which effectively grind fibrous vegetation into a pulp. The horse also developed a flexible upper lip and mobile nostrils to assist in the selection and gathering of food.

Feeding behaviour

Domesticated horses have an inbuilt feeding behaviour designed to equip them to survive. This behaviour is well developed and highly motivated and if our stable management does not allow the horse to follow this behaviour problems are likely to occur. In the wild, the horse would spend up to 60% of each 24-hour period eating; in other words, the horse is programmed to browse and graze for most of the time. Horses usually graze for up to 16 hours out of the 24, rarely going for more than 3 hours without eating. Most grazing horses sleep and relax between 1 and 6 o'clock in the morning. A study of

Camargue horses showed that they spent 30% (over 7 hours) of their time resting, either standing up or lying down. Horses only sleep 'properly' when they are lying down, usually totalling about $2\frac{1}{2}$ hours a day taken in short periods.

Horses and ponies kept in paddocks do not appear to change the time spent eating, regardless of the amount of grass available. Even if the grazing is sparse the horse will not eat for more than 60–70% of the day; conversely, an abundance of food does not 'fill the horse up' and stop it grazing. It would appear that Nature intended the horse to get fat in the spring and summer when the grass is more abundant and nutritious, to lay down reserves for the winter. During the cold weather the grass provides bulk but little feed value and the horse loses weight, ready to start the cycle again in the spring. Incidentally, this is why the wild horse is unlikely to succumb to laminitis (see 'Laminitis', Chapter 13).

Eating meat versus plants

The reason the wild horse has to spend so much time eating is that, compared with meat, plant material contains little energy and protein and much fibre. Thus, the lion can eat its fill every 2 or 3 days and sleep the rest of the time! Studies of free-living ponies have shown that they feed and range at the same level of activity both day and night. However, there is more night grazing in the summer when the heat and flies are less worrisome. Horses have mobile lips which select and gather the blades of grass together. The grass is cropped close to the ground using the incisor teeth (Fig. 1.1). While grazing horses only take a couple of mouthfuls before moving forward, one step at a time. It is estimated that they cover about 8 km (5 miles) a day as they graze.

The practical significance of this to the horse owner is that eating is psychologically and physically very important to the horse. As the amount of roughage in the diet decreases, less time is spent eating. Concentrate feeds increase leisure time and the stabled horse will spend its time displaying signs of boredom and inactivity, such as crib-biting, weaving, wind-sucking, box-walking and a whole range of 'stable vices'. This is hardly surprising since the horse was not designed to live in a stable.

Another factor to consider is that the meat-eater is eating a balanced

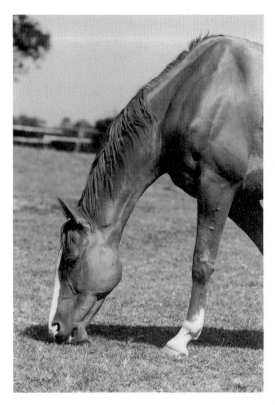

Fig. 1.1 Horses graze by cropping the grass off close to the ground with their incisor teeth.

diet which contains everything needed to sustain the body in the correct proportions. The nutritional value of vegetation will vary depending on many things, for example, time of year, type of plant, the soil it was grown on and the weather. The horse is designed to eat many different species of grasses, shrubs and herbs in order to obtain the range of nutrients required for health. If a full range of plants is not available to the horse it will not receive a balanced diet and may suffer from nutrient deficiencies. Horses grazing small, cultivated paddocks are unlikely to have access to a wide variety of grasses and herbs.

In the wild, the horse is free to roam over a wide area, the boundaries dictated by mountain ranges or rivers. Indeed, during evolution, the ancestors of the horse migrated all over the world. Herds of feral horses tend to stay in one area until they have eaten down the grass before moving on. This means that they never have to graze around their own droppings and the parasitic worm burden is kept at an acceptably low level. As they move on to new pastures the ranges of plants will gradually change depending on the geography of the area. This gradual change allows the horse's gut to acclimatise to the new diet without digestive upset. The change in diet also ensures that the horse receives the ranges of nutrients it needs.

Selection of food

While the time spent feeding does not alter much, the way in which the horse feeds may. In the summer, horses will browse on hedges and trees. In the winter, browsing may increase dramatically, depending on how hungry the horse is. Horses tend to show a preference for trees such as poplar, ash, rowan and beech and will often de-bark them (Fig. 1.2).

Horses select food using smell, taste, texture and acquired liking. When pasture has a wide variety of forage, horses will first eat what they prefer, leaving less palatable species. This means that you frequently see horse paddocks full of weeds and less palatable grasses. Several studies have shown that horses readily eat about ten species of grass. They avoid some poisonous plants but not all of them. For example, they will eat acorns, buttercups, ragwort and bracken, all of which are poisonous to horses.

Contrary to popular belief, horses are not capable of correcting a specific mineral deficiency; they do not select a mixture rich in the deficient mineral even when offered it. However, the deficient horse may develop a depraved appetite, eating soil for example. The exception to this is salt, and a horse that is deficient in salt will seek out feed rich in salt.

Horses do not like grazing round their droppings and over a period of time overgrazed paddocks tend to develop 'roughs' and 'lawns'. The lawns are closely grazed areas of preferred grasses while the roughs consist of weeds and long, rank grass. Horses use these roughs as lavatory areas, leaving the lawn to deposit their droppings and then returning to it to graze. If paddock management is poor up to half the grazing area can be lost to roughs, contaminated with droppings and carrying a heavy burden of worm eggs and larvae.

The horse is designed to thrive on a constant intake of a high fibre,

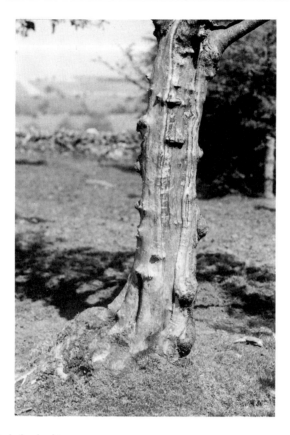

Fig. 1.2   A de-barked tree.

low nutrient diet and judging by how fat and well the average zebra looks, it is a very effective system. In summary, the horse naturally requires:

- Sixteen hours a day eating
- High fibre, low nutrient feeds
- A wide choice of vegetation
- A large area to roam
- Steady exercise.

The modern horse

The domesticated horse lives in an artificial world created by humans. Consider the changes we have made to its life style: the stabled, fit horse may have its eating reduced to three feeds and two haynets a day, perhaps only taking 5 or 6 hours to eat. It is confined to a stable often for 23 hours a day. If it is lucky enough to be turned out in the field it is still a confined area which forces the horse to graze next to its droppings. Its choice of food is taken away from it and it can only eat or drink what we offer, regardless of its quality and nutrient value. Thus we have:

- Reduced eating time
- Provided low fibre, high starch feeds
- Reduced the choice of feed
- Confined the feeding area
- Enforced idleness.

In fact, if we had set out to create the management system most likely to upset the horse we could not have done better. It is no wonder the horse develops stable vices, behavioural problems and is prone to digestive upsets.

As long as a stabled horse has access to a constant supply of roughage it will behave in a similar way to the horse at grass, spending about 60% of the time eating. However, it will not be able to socialise

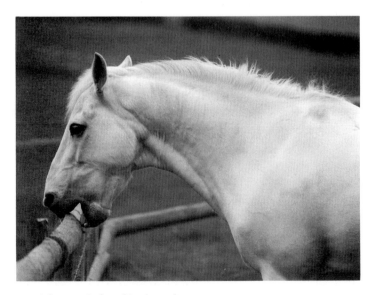

Fig. 1.3   A horse wind-sucking on a fence.

with other horses and will thus spend more time resting. Unfortunately, the horse may be reluctant to lie down in a confined space and spend little time in deep sleep. There appears to be a direct link between the restriction of feeding time and the development of stable vices, such as wind-sucking (Fig. 1.3). However, if we adopt a management and feeding system that most closely resembles the natural life style of the horse we should be able to minimise these problems.

Chapter 2
The Digestive System

Our fore-fathers realised the inherent difficulties in feeding horses and developed the 'rules of good feeding' as guidelines for all horse owners, to help them feed horses safely and effectively.

'Rules of good feeding'

All Pony Club children are able to recite at least ten rules of good feeding, but how often do we stop to consider the meaning of these rules and whether or not they still apply to the modern horse owner? Some of these 'golden rules' are listed below:

- Feed according to work, condition and temperament.
- Feed only good quality feedstuffs.
- Feed plenty of roughage.
- Feed little and often.
- Make any changes gradually.
- Keep to the same feeding time every day.
- Feed something succulent every day.
- Leave 1 hour after feeding before work.
- Water before feeding.
- Keep utensils clean.
- Reduce the amount of feed on the horse's day off.

It is worth explaining these rules in the light of modern scientific knowledge, particularly the anatomy of the digestive system.

Anatomy of the digestive system

The digestive system of the horse consists of four main areas (Fig. 2.1):

- Mouth and teeth

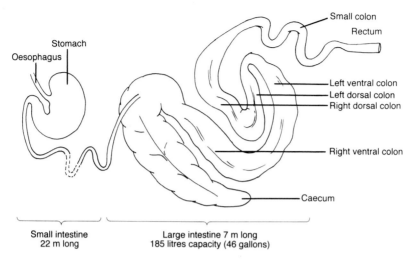

Fig. 2.1 Anatomy of the digestive system.

- Stomach
- Small intestine
- Large intestine.

As we talk about these areas some of the rules of good feeding will be explained and some ideas that perhaps should be 'rules' will come to light.

The mouth and teeth (Fig. 2.2)

Horses have a very strong, mobile and sensitive upper lip which, along with the sharp incisor teeth, enables them to bite off pieces of food in a selective fashion and graze a pasture very closely. A horse uses its lips to sift out any unpalatable ingredients of the feed, for example cubes, wormers or medications.

The tongue then moves the food to the molar teeth which pulverise the food into pieces less than 2 mm in length before swallowing. The idea is to prepare the food for digestion in the small intestine. This means that, compared with other grazing animals, the horse takes small amounts of feed at each bite and chews it slowly and carefully. This will take much longer for hay than for concentrates, taking about 1000 jaw sweeps to chew 1 kg (2.2 lb) concentrate feed and more than 3000 chews to get through the same amount of hay. This means that 1

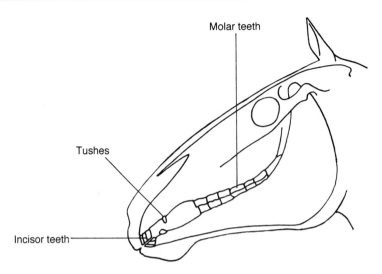

Fig. 2.2   Skull and teeth.

kg (2.2 lb) hay will keep the horse occupied for much longer than the same weight of concentrate feed. Ponies tend to chew even more thoroughly than horses, which may reflect their ability to survive on poor quality, fibrous food.

During this chewing, saliva is produced which acts to wet and lubricate the food so that it is turned into an easily swallowed 'porridge'. Saliva contains bicarbonate which is alkaline and helps counteract or 'buffer' the acid produced by the horse's stomach. If the food requires little chewing smaller amounts of saliva are produced and the food may not be properly neutralised in the stomach. This may result in poor digestion, excessive gas production and colic. Thorough chewing is essential to ensure effective digestion of the food; the addition of chaff to a concentrate feed makes good sense as it encourages more thorough chewing of each mouthful. A new rule of feeding could be:

- Always add some form of bulk, for example chaff, to a concentrate feed to prevent the horse bolting its feed and to ensure thorough chewing.

Tooth care

Efficient digestion begins with effective chewing and routine attention to the horse's teeth is an important aspect of feeding management. We have bred the horse so that it no longer has the coarse head of Przewalski's horse, but has the refined jaw and narrow nose of the Arab or Thoroughbred. This means that the top jaw is considerably wider than the bottom jaw (Fig. 2.3). The horse's teeth grow continuously; as there is incomplete overlap of the cheek teeth or molars, this means that sharp edges develop on the outside of the top cheek teeth and on the inside of the bottom cheek teeth. These sharp edges can lacerate the tongue and cheeks, making eating painful.

Sharp edges

The signs of sharp edges are:

- Quidding or dropping half-chewed food out of the mouth.
- Very slow eating.
- Excessive slobbering.
- Resistance to the bit, from altered head carriage to tossing the head or pulling hard.
- Loss of condition.
- Bolting the feed.
- Presence of whole grains or long pieces of hay in the droppings.

You can test for sharp edges by pressing on the sides of the horse's face, along the teeth edges. The horse may show discomfort or pull away if the teeth are sharp. Any lean horse that is failing to gain condition despite being wormed and being fed a better diet should have its teeth checked.

The vet or horse dentist can rasp or float these sharp edges and a horse's teeth should be checked a twice a year and rasped if necessary. Horses on a hay and concentrate ration tend to develop sharp edges sooner than ponies or horses kept at grass. Checking the horse's teeth should begin once the horse starts to lose its milk teeth ($2\frac{1}{2}$ years of age). It is also wise to have the teeth checked before introducing the bit to the young horse; if the horse's mouth is sore it is much more likely to resent being mouthed (having the bit introduced). It is also sensible to check the horse's incisor teeth for signs of abnormal wear as this may indicate that the horse is a wind-sucker or crib-biter.

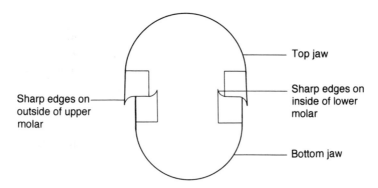

Fig. 2.3 The overlap in a horse's teeth.

The stomach

The horse's stomach lies under the diaphragm (Fig. 2.4), separated from the gullet by a muscular ring called the cardiac sphincter which is so powerful that it can be regarded as a one-way valve, not allowing regurgitation of gas or food. Thus, the horse cannot vomit, and excess

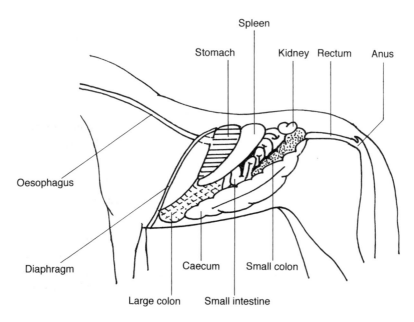

Fig. 2.4 The position of the stomach and abdominal organs in relation to the diaphragm.

gas production in the stomach cannot be relieved by burping and may result in serious colic.

The horse is a grazing animal; it evolved to be a 'trickle feeder' with a gut designed to cope with the regular intake of small quantities of fibrous food. The most important thing to remember is that the small size of the horse's stomach results in the horse's desire to feed almost continuously. This is the reason for the rule of good feeding which everybody remembers best – feed little and often.

The horse's stomach when empty is less than 10% of the total gut volume, about 8 l (1.7 gallons) in a 16-hh (hands; 162-cm) horse, about the size of a rugby ball. The stomach can stretch to accommodate about 18 l (4 gallons), but the 'J' shape of the stomach means that it is never more than two-thirds full (Fig. 2.5). In other words, the horse's stomach will hold about 12 l (2.5 gallons), about two-thirds of a standard water bucket.

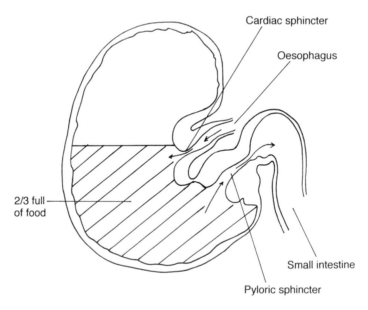

Fig. 2.5   The 'J' shape of the horse's stomach.

Allowing for the quantity of saliva the horse produces, the best meal size is limited to just over half a bucketful. Feeding any more than this is wasteful as the horse cannot digest it efficiently and it may even cause colic. Stabled horses should be fed at least twice a day and performance horses on larger concentrate rations should be fed three or four times a day.

A full stomach puts pressure on the diaphragm, the muscular sheet which separates the lungs and the guts, preventing the horse from filling its lungs effectively. However, most of a feed will have passed into the small intestine after about 45 minutes, hence the rule 'do not work fast for at least 1 hour after feeding'. Liquids pass rapidly through the stomach and little of the water a horse drinks during or after a feed mixes with the stomach contents. It is more useful to ensure that the horse has a 'constant supply of fresh, clean water' than it is to 'water before feeding'. As a rule, the grazing horse will only take a long drink once or twice a day (see 'Rules of watering', Chapter 9). There is relatively little digestion of food in the stomach, but the acid stomach secretions physically break down the feed and kill any bacteria that may have been ingested.

The small intestine

The small intestine is a tube running from the stomach to the large intestine, and the total length is about 21 m (70 ft) with a capacity of about 30 l (6.6 gallons). The small intestine can move quite freely except at its attachment to the stomach and caecum; it lies in numerous coils in conjunction with the small colon. Food particles travel quite rapidly through the small intestine, the majority of the food taking only 60 minutes to reach the large intestine.

Secretions from the pancreas (pancreatic juice) and liver (bile) combine with secretions from the small intestine to digest soluble carbohydrate (sugars and starches), protein and fat. The small intestine is where most of the breakdown and absorption of the concentrate part of the horse's diet takes place, using a similar process to that in the human, pig or dog. Therefore it plays an important role for the competition horse on a high concentrate diet. Under natural conditions where the horse is eating a fibrous diet of grass, the small intestine is much less important, as is reflected by the speed at which food passes through it. The speed of passage means that starch may not be effectively digested, leading to digestive complications (see 'Indigestion', Chapter 14).

Many minerals are absorbed from the small intestine including calcium, zinc, copper, manganese, iron and magnesium. Phosphorus, sodium, potassium and chloride are absorbed from both the large and small intestines. Most vitamins in the feed are absorbed from the small intestine. The remaining fibrous portion of the feed and undigested starch and protein pass on for digestion in the large intestine. The horse does not have a gall bladder in which to store bile; instead bile trickles continuously into the small intestine. This serves to remind us that the horse evolved as a trickle feeder, needing frequent, small feeds. Horses appear to be good at digesting fat and vegetable fat is often added to horse's diets.

The large intestine

So far what we have read is very similar to that of the digestive processes of the dog, pig or indeed human. However, we would look very thin on a diet of grass. What allows the horse to thrive on a feed that would not nourish us? The answer lies in the horse's hind gut or large intestine, which is able to extract the energy locked up in the tough, fibrous part of plants. Like us, the horse does not have any digestive enzymes that are capable of breaking down the fibre that makes up plant cell walls; however, certain bacteria can break it down by a fermentation process. Unlike us, the horse has a greatly enlarged large intestine, making up 60% of the total gut volume. This huge gut houses a vast number of micro-organisms which release energy from the fibre in the horse's diet by fermentation.

The large intestine is about 8 m (25 ft) long and consists of four parts:

- Caecum
- Large colon
- Small colon
- Rectum.

The caecum is a large, blind-ended sac lying on the floor of the abdomen. The large colon is about 3 m (10 ft) long and in order to fit into the horse's abdomen it has to fold into four regions; the points where the colon narrows and turns are vulnerable to blockage. If for any reason the passage of digesta through the colon is slowed down, obstruction and hence colic may occur. The job of the large intestine is the microbial digestion of fibre. The large intestine houses millions of bacteria and other micro-organisms which 'feed' on the fibre, fermenting it, to release substances useful to the horse. Thus, in return for a cosy, warm environment with plenty of food, the bacteria and other micro-organisms break down the fibre in the horse's diet into a form which can be used by the horse as a source of energy.

The large intestine is only held in place in the abdomen by its bulk; if the gut is too empty problems may arise because the gut is more able to move about. This brings us to another rule of feeding – feed plenty of bulk. If the gut is to be healthy and efficient the horse should receive at least half its ration as roughage, even if it is in hard, fast work.

The numbers and types of bacteria in the gut are dependent on the type of ration being fed; it is important to maintain a continuous supply of a consistent diet so that the population of bacteria is in a steady state. The bacteria and other micro-organisms are very fussy and any change in their surroundings, such as a sudden change in what the horse is eating, kills them. This may result in digestive upsets, such as the horse scouring (diarrhoea or loose droppings) and losing condition, hence the rule *'make any changes to the diet gradually'*.

The benefits to the horse of housing these bacteria and other micro-organisms are threefold:

- Digestion of otherwise unavailable fibre
- The manufacture of B vitamins and vitamin K
- The manufacture of essential amino acids and protein.

The bacteria themselves consist of a high percentage of protein, but it is not known how much of this can be utilised by the horse. This means that horses, particularly youngstock, need good quality protein (see 'Protein quality', Chapter 3).

The physiology of digestion

The digestive processes that take place in the horse are different from those in other grass-eaters such as the cow, which is a ruminant. In the horse, easily digested food material is first broken down by digestive enzymes in the small intestine. Only insoluble material reaches the large intestine for bacterial fermentation. This insoluble material is mainly cellulose. In the wild the horse is a trickle feeder, eating a mainly fibrous diet and this is very efficient; in an all-hay diet, over 70% of the horse's energy is derived from hind-gut digestion.

Stabled horses tend to be given three feeds a day; this food passes rapidly through the gut and there is often insufficient time for all the soluble material to be completely digested by the enzymes in the small intestine. Remaining soluble material passes into the caecum which not only is wasteful but also can cause severe digestive upset (see 'Indigestion', Chapter 14). Even feeding a horse more than three times a day will lead to fluctuations in the conditions in the large intestine and potential digestive upset. Ideally horses should receive uniform, 'complete' diets where each mouthful throughout the day provides the same nutrients, just as the feral grazing horse would experience. In practice, even stabling horses at night and feeding them hay, then turning them out to grass during the day will alter the conditions within the gut. We can help this situation by feeding fibre in the form of chaff with the concentrate feed and giving the horse probiotics in times of stress (See 'Probiotics', Chapter 14). As the competition horse is fed more concentrates, more emphasis is placed on digestion in the small intestine and there is a case for increasing the protein and vitamin content of the feed to compensate for the loss of nutrients from the gut bacteria and other micro-organisms.

Chapter 3
Staying Alive: Nutrients and Nutrient Requirements

Just as a yoghurt pot or chocolate bar tells you the nutritional value of the food you are eating, so feed companies have to declare the nutrient content of cubes and mixes made for horses on the bag of feed (Fig. 3.1). When you are deciding which feed to buy it helps to know what these figures mean.

The feeds that we give to horses are often grouped into basic sources of:

- Energy
- Protein
- Fat
- Fibre.

Most feeds contain a combination of all of these things, and also provide various amounts of minerals and vitamins. To stay healthy, horses need a balanced, daily supply of these nutrients along with fresh, clean water.

Energy

Horses need energy to stay alive, to fuel the on-going body processes and to maintain their body temperature. They also need extra energy to:

- Grow
- Reproduce
- Recover from illness
- Work.

SUPER CHAFF

This is a complementary feeding stuff with molasses for horses and ponies.

Total sugar (as sucrose)	20.00%	Crude ash	19.00%
Crude protein	6.00%	Moisture	22.00%
Crude fibre	19.00%	Estimated digestible energy	9.5 MJ/kg

Ingredients: molasses, feed quality barley/oat straw, hay, limestone flour, seaweed, salt.

Introduce the chaff gradually, building up to your horse's requirement. This is a non-heating food stuff and can therefore be fed in any amount you wish.

(a)

COMPETITION CUBES

Ideal non-heating cubes for horses in regular and competition work and needing more energy:

Protein	11.5%	Fibre	12.0%
Oil	3.25%	Digestible energy	11.0 MJ/kg

- Non-heating
- For horses and ponies in regular and competition work
- For putting condition on poor horses

(b)

Fig. 3.1 Example of a declaration of ingredients on (a) a bag of chaff, (b) a bag of cubes.

Calorie counting for horses

We are all familiar with the concept of counting the calories in food when dieting. High calorie foods are fattening, they contain more energy than we can burn up and the excess is laid down as fat. High calorie foods include sugar, starch (carbohydrates) and fat. When we are looking at the energy value of feeds for horses we use the metric version of the calorie, the joule (J). To make the figures easier, the term megajoules of digestible energy per kilogram is used (MJ DE/kg). Thus, a high energy food like oats may contain up to 14 MJ DE/kg, while a low energy feed like grass hay may only contain 7 MJ DE/kg, half as much as oats. Concentrates contain higher levels of energy than forages, hence their name.

Carbohydrates

Energy is available to the horse in several different forms, including fat, carbohydrate and protein. Energy can also be obtained by using body reserves in the liver, muscles and fat deposits. Carbohydrates are traditionally the main source of energy, with 'heating' feeds such as oats and barley containing high energy levels. Traditionally these have been fed to working horses to provide them with the energy to do the work demanded of them. More recently cubes and mixes have also been used to provide the horse with energy. There are two types of carbohydrate: soluble and insoluble.

Soluble carbohydrate

Soluble carbohydrates consist of starches and sugars. They are present in large amounts in spring grass, cereals and most cubes and mixes. Starches and sugars are broken down in the small intestine by the action of the digestive enzymes. The result of this breakdown is sugar or glucose which is then absorbed through the gut wall, into the bloodstream. From here it can either be used as a fuel to provide the energy needed to drive muscles or stored for later use. We can get an instant burst of energy by drinking a glucose drink; this does not demand any digestion, but can pass straight into the blood, replenishing our blood sugar levels. High starch foods such as oats and barley are rapidly digested in the small intestine providing the horse with 'instant energy'; this burst of energy may be one of the reasons why cereal grains can have a 'heating' effect on a horse's temperament.

Insoluble carbohydrate

Insoluble carbohydrate makes up a large proportion of the natural diet of the horse; it is the cellulose and fibre found in grass and hay. Fibre is not broken down to any great extent in the small intestine but passes to the large intestine where it is acted on by the gut bacteria and other micro-organisms to provide an energy source for the horse. The energy from the breakdown and fermentation of fibre is released more slowly; this steady supply of 'slow release energy' is much more natural for the horse. Remember, the horse is designed to eat fibre not starch and keeping starch levels down will result in a happier, healthier horse.

Too much carbohydrate

If the horse is fed too much energy there will be serious consequences:

- Receiving too much energy can make the horse almost hyperactive. All that energy is being released into the horse's system and it only has the four walls of its stable to look at. No wonder it thinks dressage is a waste of time.
- As we know only too well, if you eat too much the excess is stored as fat. Horses, like us, are less athletic if they are overweight, and working fat horses strains muscles, tendons and joints.
- More seriously, too much carbohydrate can affect the horse's metabolism; a carbohydrate overload resulting from rich spring grass or stealing from the feed bin can lead to laminitis.

Starch digestion

Starch is a complex substance, made of many glucose segments bound together. If the horse is receiving a large amount of concentrate feed, it can be a problem for the horse to break down the starch in the short time that it is in the small intestine. Starch will then pass into the large intestine where it is rapidly fermented by the micro-organisms. This upsets the delicate balance in the hind gut, leading to acid conditions which in turn can result in severe conditions such as colic and laminitis. The cooked starch found in extruded and micronised feeds is much easier for the horse to deal with.

Energy requirements for maintenance

The energy requirement of a horse that is not working is known as the horse's maintenance requirement. The energy required for maintenance is proportional to the horse's bodyweight. This should not really be a surprise; larger horses need more food to stay alive than smaller ponies. The maintenance requirement will be affected by:

- Temperament
- Time of year
- Weather conditions

- Shelter available
- Type or breed of horse.

As a guideline, horses and ponies at rest can maintain their bodyweight with an amount of feed equal to about 1.5-2% of their bodyweight. This is shown in Table 3.1. The lower hay figure is for the lighter animal that is a good-doer (puts on condition easily); the larger hay figure is for the heavier horse that is a poor-doer (does not make good use of its feed). Most horses will maintain their bodyweight on a hay ration that is somewhere between the two figures. Thus, if you had a 16 hh (162-cm) horse on box rest (24 hours enforced rest in the stable due to injury or illness) it would need about 10 kg (22 lb) hay per day to satisfy its energy requirements. This is likely to be less than the horse wants to eat, which is why inactive horses tend to put on weight.

Table 3.1   Relationship between height, bodyweight and maintenance requirement.

Height		Bodyweight		Ration of medium quality hay per day	
(hh)	(cm)	(kg)	(lb)	(kg)	(lb)
11	111	200–260	440–572	3–5	6.6–11
12	122	230–290	506–638	3.5–6	7.7–13.2
13	132	290–350	638–770	4.5–7	9.9–15.4
14	142	350–420	770–924	5.5–8.5	12.1–18.7
15	152	420–520	924–1144	6.5–10.5	14.3–23.1
16	162	500–600	1100–1320	8–12	17.6–26.4
17	172	600–725	1320–1595	9–14	19.8–30.8

Energy requirements for work

The energy required by the individual horse for work is influenced by:

- The speed and duration of the work
- The terrain, i.e. hilly or rough
- The weather conditions, i.e. temperature and humidity
- The horse's condition and fitness
- The horse's conformation and soundness

- The ability of the rider; it is harder work carrying an unbalanced rider
- The horse's temperament.

This means that no two horses will have the same energy requirement and the ration will have to be adjusted to suit the individual animal. Highly strung horses may expend twice as much energy as more placid horses doing the same work. These horses also tend to fret in their stables, further increasing their energy requirement. As these horses are often fed less in an attempt to contain their temperament they are often very difficult to keep in good condition. It has been estimated that galloping uses up twice as much energy as trotting and five times as much energy as walking. The weight of the rider should also be taken into consideration; a horse carrying a heavy burden will use up more energy than one with a light, balanced rider.

The horse has a limit to its appetite, in other words how much it can eat every day. Therefore as the demand for energy increases the proportion of low energy, bulk feeds has to fall and the proportion of high energy, concentrate feed has to increase. Hay, even fed to appetite, will not supply all the energy demands of a galloping racehorse. A high roughage diet also tends to give the horse a large belly; reducing the bulk in the diet allows the horse to develop the trim outline required by the athlete.

Fibre levels

Remembering the rule of good feeding – feed plenty of bulk, the fibre level in the ration should not fall below 50%. An adequate level of fibre is essential to maintain the flow of food through the gut. Fibre also tends to open out the digestive mixture, allowing the digestive juices to act on the feed more efficiently. Additionally, fibre helps to retain water and electrolytes in the large intestine, acting as a reservoir of fluid for the working, sweating horse.

Fat

Fat is a concentrated source of energy. What are first things the human weight watcher has to cut out? Cream, butter, cheese and chocolate, all high in fat. Fat contains two-and-a-quarter times as much energy as the equivalent amount of carbohydrate. Traditionally horse diets contained about 2–3% fat. Over recent years cubes and mixes have been formulated with higher oil levels and vegetable oil has been added to rations to supply extra energy. Horses are good at digesting fat and it provides energy in a 'non-heating' form and is unlikely to cause temperament upsets.

As fat is so energy dense, the horse will not have to eat as much food to meet its energy needs. This is very useful for horses with poor appetites or those that do not 'do' well. Horses will eat corn oil, sunflower oil and soya oil. Blended vegetable oils, although cheaper, are probably best avoided as you cannot be sure what they consist of. Cod liver oil is fed as a vitamin supplement, not an energy source; it does not fulfil the same role as vegetable oil.

Oil should be introduced gradually into the diet, i.e. over a period of 2 weeks to a minimum of 300 ml (0.5 pt) divided equally between the horse's feeds. This is the minimum that makes its addition worthwhile and is equivalent, in energy terms, to about 900 g (2 lb) oats. Oil can be added at the rate of up to 10% of the concentrate ration; this would amount to about 600 ml (1 pt) per day.

Extra fat in the diet demands the addition of vitamin E. As a guideline, 100 iu (international unit) extra vitamin E should be supplied for every 100 ml (0.2 pt) oil. This is in addition to the horse's normal daily requirement. If substantial amounts of oil [over 300 ml (0.5 pt) per day] are used to replace grain or cubes in the ration, it may be necessary to reassess the protein and mineral requirements of the horse.

Protein

Protein makes up body tissue and horses that have a high protein requirement include:

- Growing youngsters
- Pregnant and lactating mares
- Horses recovering from illness.

Protein is what makes up muscle; it does not have a role in energy production unless fed in excess. The extra muscle laid down by the working horse only increases the protein requirement very slightly.

Protein quality

Proteins are made up of strings of building blocks called amino acids in much the same way that letters are strung together to make different words. There are over 20 different amino acids resulting in proteins with structures as diverse as hair and steak. Just as you need a few vital vowels to help the consonants form words, certain amino acids must be present if the horse is to make the best use of the protein in the diet. The amino acids lysine and methionine are important and proteins containing these are called good quality proteins and must be included in the horse's diet. Plant proteins tend to be of lower quality than animal proteins. Of all the vegetable proteins soya provides the horse with the best balance of amino acids.

Not all proteins are equally digestible; leather contains protein but it is not very digestible. So another important aspect of protein quality is its digestibility, i.e. how much of the protein in the feed is actually available to the horse. The crude protein gives an idea of the total amount of protein in the feed, while the digestible crude protein gives an indication of how much of that protein is available to the horse. For example, in a sample of haylage the crude protein might be 11% but the digestible crude protein is only 6.7%. The protein might be 60% digestible.

Diets that contain poor quality protein, for example an oats-and hay-based diet, must be fed in greater quantities than those containing better quality protein. Adding a good quality protein source to the diet, for example soya, will help the horse maintain condition more effectively. This is a useful point to bear in mind when feeding poor-doers or horses with small appetites. However, although excess protein can be converted into energy, overfeeding protein is an expensive way to provide energy and may even be detrimental to performance.

Protein requirements for maintenance

The adult horse needs enough protein in the diet to be able to make good any day-to-day protein losses. This amounts to about 8% crude protein in the ration. This should be supplied by good quality hay, but if the hay is of poor quality the protein levels may not be adequate. Under these circumstances the horse may lose condition even though it is eating all the hay it can. Adding soyabean meal or alfalfa to the ration will boost the protein quality.

Protein requirements are better expressed as grams per day to avoid the problem of varying protein content of different feedstuffs. For example, a 16-hh (162-cm) horse being fed average quality hay to appetite (60 g/kg or 6% crude protein) will receive about 720 g crude protein per day. Only 4 kg of a competition mix (130 g/kg or 13% crude protein) supplies 1000 g crude protein per day.

Protein requirements for work

Exercise increases the horse's daily requirement for protein as the muscle mass and red blood cell production increase. However, providing adequate energy is available there is no benefit in feeding rations containing more than 10–12% crude protein. Remember, this is the overall protein of the ration, not the protein content of the concentrate. Taking our 16-hh (162-cm) horse in hard work, receiving a ration of 50% medium quality hay (8% crude protein) and 50% concentrates, in order to push the total protein of the ration up to 10% the concentrate must provide 12% crude protein. This is why most competition feeds have quite high protein levels; they have to make up for the shortfall of protein almost always present in the hay. The energy and protein requirements of brood mares, stallions and youngstock are discussed in Chapter 15.

Chapter 4
Feeds and Feed Processing

Today there is a huge selection of feeds for the horse owner to choose from, ranging from haylage through cereal grains to a bewildering choice of cubes and coarse mixes. The aim of this chapter is to help the horse owner to make an educated decision about what to feed his or her horse.

The amount of nutrition that can be obtained from a feed depends on several factors including:

- Processing the feed. Crushing or rolling tend to increase the digestibility and palatability of feeds, allowing the horse's digestive juices to work more efficiently
- Fibre content
- Thoroughness with which the horse chews the feed
- Exercise level of the horse
- Amount of feed eaten.

Roughage

Roughage and forage are often thought to mean the same thing, but the dictionary definition of forage is food for horses and cattle. This means all types of feed. Roughage is defined as coarse fodder, the indigestible material in food which stimulates the action of the intestines. Roughage provides bulk and fibre and satisfies the horse's appetite. Roughages fed to horses include grass, hay, barn-dried hay, straw, haylage, silage, alfalfa and dried grass.

Grass

Grass is the horse's natural feed. It contains large amounts of water along with protein, fibre and water-soluble carbohydrate (sugars).

Unlike cereal grains, grass does not contain any starch; this is one of the reasons why horses on high cereal diets may experience digestive upsets – their gut is not designed to cope with starch. However, problems may arise when horses graze lush, well fertilised pastures of rich grass such as Italian ryegrass. Their intake of water-soluble carbohydrate may be so high that it is not all digested in the small intestine but passes into the hind gut, upsetting the balance of micro-organisms and causing digestive upset. In severe cases the horse or pony will suffer from laminitis.

Grass can be cut, dried and cubed as grass meal. The feeding value of grass changes throughout the year. Spring grass is lush, containing high levels of protein and sugars and a low fibre content (Fig. 4.1). As the grass ages it becomes more fibrous and less nutritious with low levels of protein and energy.

In practical terms, horses will become fat in the spring because good grass over-supplies their requirement for energy. The only way to stop this is to restrict the grazing and satisfy their appetite by feeding hay or

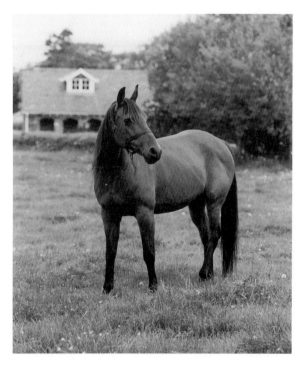

Fig. 4.1 Lush spring grass.

straw. In the winter the feeding value of grass is minimal and most horses will require supplementary feeding. Table 4.1 shows the nutrient composition of different species of grass. Old established pastures are likely to contain a mixture of grass species with little ryegrass; these pastures are more suitable for horses and are the source of meadow hay. Rich, specially seeded ryegrass leys are designed for dairy cattle, seed hay and silage crops.

Table 4.1   Nutrient composition of grasses.

Grass species	Protein (%)	Fibre (%)	Soluble carbohydrates (%)
Timothy	16	35	6
Cocksfoot	14	41	9
Fescue	13	40	6
Perennial ryegrass	18	28	16
Italian ryegrass	10–19	26–33	15–24

Hay

Hay that is properly produced and correctly stored is a valuable part of the horse's diet; poor quality hay not only means that the horse will need extra concentrates, but also can be detrimental to the horse's health. Buying cheap, poor quality hay is always false economy. The nutrient value of hay will depend on:

- The nutrient value of the grass when the hay was cut
- How efficiently the grass was dried, turned and baled.

Properties of good quality hay

- Clean, fresh and sweet-smelling
- Green
- Free from dust and mould
- Texture: meadow hay is finer and softer while seed hay is more spiky and straw-like
- Type of grasses: a ryegrass hay is potentially of a higher feed value than timothy hay
- Time of cutting: if you can identify seed heads then the grass was cut late and the hay will be of lower feed value.

Hay can meet all these criteria and still be of poor nutrient value and the only way to establish the true value of hay is to have it analysed. Before buying hay in quantity it is worth sending a sample off for laboratory analysis. This will tell you the nutrient value of the hay and the amount of fungal spores present. Most hay made in the UK is mature, stemmy and low quality. It is also likely to be deficient in protein and calcium, something that should be remembered for horses that are only being fed hay.

As far as the horse owner is concerned the most important thing is for the hay to be free of dust, mould and fungal spores. Mouldy hay can cause irreparable damage to the horse's lungs. As long as hay is clean, any deficiency can be made up by feeding concentrates or supplements. You should always buy the best quality hay you can afford.

Hay alternatives

The British climate is not ideally suited to making hay and as a result horse owners may be faced with a shortage of good quality hay, leading them to seek alternative fibre sources for their horses. The horse is designed to live on a high fibre diet; any shortfall of hay must be compensated for by adding another high fibre feed, for example:

- Silage
- Haylage
- Straw
- Chaffs
- Sugar beet pulp
- High fibre cubes
- Succulents, e.g. carrots.

Table 4.2 shows the nutrient composition of hay and some other high fibre feeds.

The proportion of bulk in the horse's diet is determined by the amount and type of work it is doing. Horses and ponies doing the majority of their work in walk and trot need very little concentrate feed while horses working at faster paces may need less bulk and more concentrates. It is unlikely that a horse in moderate work, including the occasional day's competition or hunting, would require more than one-third of the ration as concentrates.

Table 4.2 Composition of hay and other high fibre feeds.

Feed	Crude protein (%)	Crude fibre (%)	Digestible energy (MJ DE/kg)	Dry matter (%)	pH
Hay	4.5–10	30–40	7–10	80	
Silage	10	30	10	25	
Haylage	8–14	30–38	9–11.5	55–65	5.3–5.8
Straw	3	40	6	88	
Sugar beet pulp	7	34	10.5	Fed soaked	
Alfalfa chaff	15–16	32	9–10	80	
Alfalfa/straw chaff	10.5	38	7	80	
High fibre cubes	9	20	8.5	85	
Grassmeal	16	36	9–10	85	

Most of the hay alternatives mentioned have a better nutrient value than the hay they are replacing or supplementing and should be fed carefully; it may be necessary to reduce or change the concentrate ration. If a high energy forage replacer is being used it may be necessary to feed a lower energy concentrate, for example a high fibre mix or cube. This is preferable to feeding less of the same concentrate as it helps maintain the fibre levels of the ration and satisfy the horse's appetite.

If hay is replaced by a more concentrated energy source, such as haylage, the horse will eat its day's ration of food more quickly and may be come bored, developing stable vices such as crib-biting or wind-sucking. Boredom is less likely to be a problem, for example, in the busy riding school horse than in the livery animal which is only ridden for an hour a day. All new feeds, including hay alternatives such as haylage, straw and silage, should be introduced gradually into the horse's ration to avoid digestive upset.

Silage and haylage

Silage is grass preserved by pickling it in its own juices. The grass is cut much earlier than for hay and silage is therefore highly nutritious. Well-made silage is virtually dust and fungal spore-free; however, feeding silage is often not a practical proposition for horse owners for two reasons:

- Silage is made in silos, clamps or big bales; these methods pose considerable logistical problems – how do you get the silage to the horse? Bales start to deteriorate 3 or 4 days after they are opened which means that 12–14 horses are needed to use a bale without wastage, based on an intake of 10 kg (22 lb) silage per day.
- The packaging and storage of silage are vital; if done incorrectly potentially lethal micro-organisms can develop. Always examine the packaging carefully; if the bags are punctured or split there may be potentially fatal spoilage.

Haylage (Fig. 4.2) lies between silage and hay in its feeding value and digestibility. It is highly palatable and horses can take in large amounts of energy quite rapidly so care should be taken not to overfeed. Haylage should be substituted for hay on a weight for weight basis; it contains a lot of water and is consequently heavy, so that the horse will be receiving equivalent amounts of energy and protein from a smaller volume ration. The downside of this is that the horse will be receiving less fibre and the haylage will be eaten more quickly than the equivalent hay ration.

Before buying silage or haylage find out how it was made and have it analysed to assess the quality. Consider the following points:

- Amounts of nitrogen used on the grass
- Period between last nitrogen application and cutting (this should be 10 weeks for horses)
- No preservatives should have been used in the making of the silage or haylage
- Look, smell and feel (should be like slightly damp hay with the consistency of tobacco and a pleasant smell).

Apart from the nutritional value an analysis will show the quality of the fermentation that has taken place. Correct fermentation is vital to preserve the silage or haylage and also affects its suitability for feeding to horses. The following guidelines should be used:

- The dry matter should be between 45 and 65%, preferably 55–65%; however, forage with a dry matter of only 45% can be considered if all the other parameters are satisfactory.

- The pH (acidity) should lie between 4.5 and 5.8. Silage or hay-lage with a pH of less than 4.5 is often unpalatable and may cause scouring; it can also be fatal to donkeys. Above a pH of 6 the silage or haylage will not be acidic enough to prevent the potentially lethal micro-organisms developing.
- The ammonia nitrogen level should be less than 5%.

Very early or late cut silage or haylage may fall outside these para-meters and should be used carefully.

Some haylage is also produced specifically for horses. Grass is cut and allowed to wilt until the moisture content is down to about 45% and then baled in the same way as hay. The bales are then compressed to about half their size and sealed in tough, plastic bags. Fermentation takes place which preserves the grass. Different types of bagged hay-lage are produced, for example alfalfa and high fibre types are avail-able. Special closely woven haynets (Fig. 4.3) can be used to feed haylage in order to slow down the horse's rate of eating.

Straw

Good quality straw in small quantities can act as a useful source of fibre for horses with sound teeth, but it is deficient in most nutrients. Straw is useful to feed as bulk to accompany a haylage- or silage-based ration. It is also a good filler for fat ponies that do too well on hay. Care must be taken to provide correct levels of minerals and vitamins if straw is to be used in the diet. Straw can also be used with dried grass or dried alfalfa. Equal proportions of straw and alfalfa are equivalent to feeding an average quality hay. Hungry horses brought in onto straw beds may eat too much straw which can lead to impactive colic (see Chapter 13).

Chaffs

Most straw-based, molassed chaffs are designed to bulk out the hard feed (concentrate ration) and to slow down the horse's rate of eating. They generally have a low protein content and are not really suitable as a hay replacer. Hay and alfalfa or straw chaffs have been designed as partial or complete hay replacers, to be fed pound for pound for good quality hay. A version has even been specially formulated for laminitic horses and ponies. However, they tend to work out even more

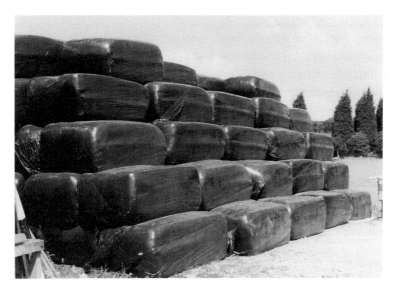

Fig. 4.2   Haylage bales.

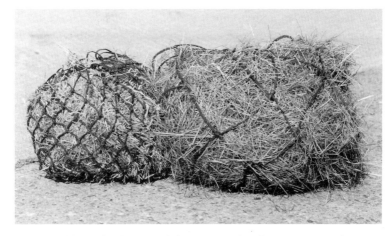

Fig. 4.3   Small hole haylage net (left), compared with a conventional net.

expensive than the most expensive hay. Alfalfa chaff is too 'high-powered' to be fed to most horses as a hay replacer, but is a useful 'top-up', especially for horses in hard work, being high in energy, protein, minerals and vitamins. A useful fibre-provider for the older horse which finds chewing hay a problem is a mixture of alfalfa pellets soaked with sugar beet pulp.

Sugar beet pulp

The high digestible fibre content of sugar beet pulp means that it is a compromise between a roughage and a concentrate. It should be soaked overnight for feeding the following day to prevent it swelling in the horse's gut. Sufficient water should be used to create a damp, crumbly texture; there is no point in having a sloppy feed and losing nutrients in unused liquid. This also allows the horse to take in a larger quantity of beet pulp without filling up on water. Horses can be fed up to 1.8 kg (4 lb) dry weight of beet pulp per day; this amounts to about 4 scoops of wet sugar beet pulp and would replace 1.8 kg (4 lb) hay. Sugar beet pulp is also a useful source of calcium. Un-molassed sugar beet pulp is now available, reducing the soluble carbohydrate level of the diet.

High fibre cubes

Most high fibre cubes are not designed to replace the entire hay ration; however, they can be used to supplement poor quality grazing and they can be added to the ration when hay is in short supply. It is not recommended that more than one-third of the hay ration is replaced by high fibre cubes; in practical terms this amounts to about 4 kg (9 lb) for a 16-hh (162-cm) horse. The cubes should be fed in at least four feeds a day if they are being used to replace part of the hay ration. This is partly to prevent the horse becoming bored and partly for digestive efficiency. High fibre cubes are also useful to maintain the condition of resting horses and ponies and those suddenly thrown out of work, when they can replace the concentrate ration.

Succulents

Succulents such as carrots and swedes are useful for adding variety to the diet and to help alleviate the boredom factor. It is not recommended that more than 2 kg (4 lb) per day is fed. Potatoes should be avoided.

Energy concentrates

As the horse's workload increases 'hard' feed or concentrates are added to the diet and the proportion of hay reduced. Before the arrival of compound cubes and coarse mixes horse owners relied on 'straights' to provide the horse with energy and protein – horse diets were based on oats and bran with barley, peas and beans added when necessary. Despite the popularity of compound feeds, straights still play an important role in feeding horses. Table 4.3 describes the appearance, nutritional value and feeding hints for some energy sources for horses. Maize, oats, naked oats, wheat and barley are cereals suitable for feeding to horses. Sorghum, rye and rice are also used as energy sources in some countries. Extruded wheat is used in some coarse mixes to add a palatable source of energy.

Table 4.3   Appearance, nutritional value and feeding hints for some energy sources.

Feed	Description	Nutritional value	Feeding hints
Oats	Plump, shiny, clean, dust-free. Can be fed whole or crimped	8–13% crude protein 11–14 MJ DE/kg 10–12% fibre 4.5% oil Low in calcium, B complex vitamins, vitamin A and lysine	Palatable, easily digested, 'safer' to feed than other cereals, high in fibre, low in energy, weigh light. Can make up all the concentrate ration. Avoid 'new' oats (less than 3 months old)
Naked oats	Oats without the husk	13% crude protein 16 MJ DE/kg 3% fibre 9% oil	Energy-dense. Good for performance horses with poor appetites
Barley	Plump, dust-free, rounder than oats. Fed rolled, steam flaked, micronised or boiled. Cooked barley is more digestible and less likely to lead to starch overload	8–10% crude protein 12–13 MJ DE/kg 5% fibre 2% oil Low in calcium, B complex vitamins, vitamin A and lysine	Provides more energy and lower fibre than oats and weighs heavier. Some horses are allergic to it; cooking may solve this problem. Can make up all the concentrate ration

Contd

Table 4.3 contd

Feed	Description	Nutritional value	Feeding hints
Maize (Fig. 4.4)	Can be fed whole, but usually steam flaked and rolled	8% crude protein 14–15 MJ DE/kg 3% fibre 4% oil	Most energy-dense grain, palatable and digestible. Useful for poor-doers or horses with very high energy requirements. Not usually more than 25% of the concentrate ration
Bran	By-product of flour production. Should be free-flowing, fluffy flakes with little dust. May be fed as mash; however, not a good laxative as once claimed	15% crude protein 10 MJ DE/kg 11% fibre 3% oil Not very high in fibre. Low in calcium	Platable, weighs very light. Expensive, largely replaced by chaffs. No more than 10% of the concentrate ration
Oil	Sunflower, corn and soya oils are preferred	0% crude protein 35 MJ DE/kg 0% fibre Very good energy source. Cod liver oil provides vitamins A, D and E and essential fatty acids	Minimum of 300 ml (0.5 pt) vegetable oil per day up to 1 l (1.75 pt). Increases vitamin E requirement. 300 ml (0.5 pt) replaces 900 g (2 lb) oats

Cereals

Cereals are good sources of energy. The majority of the energy is present as starch and, as discussed in Chapter 2 'The small intestine', large feeds can result in undigested starch passing through the small intestine and into the large intestine. Rapid fermentation in the large intestine can upset the delicate balance of micro-organisms, leading to digestive upset. In most cases this will not result in laminitis or serious metabolic problems, but may well contribute to the 'heating' effect of cereals and temperament changes. Cereals are deficient in calcium and a diet based on cereals will need a limestone supplement to correct the calcium-to-phosphorus ratio. Cereals tend to have only moderate protein levels and when fed with average quality hay there may not be enough protein in the ration.

Cereal grains are often fed rolled or crimped. Adult horses with good teeth that chew their food thoroughly should be able to cope with whole oats. However, rolling is useful for foals, old horses and greedy horses that bolt their feed. If the grains are not being chewed and hence digested properly, whole grains will appear in the droppings. Once grain has been rolled the kernel is exposed to the air and the feed value will start to fall. Always buy from a supplier that has a rapid turnover of stock to try to ensure that the bags have not been standing for a long time. Do not buy too much at one time; buying more frequently will ensure fresh feed.

Protein concentrates

Horses need protein for growth, work and during pregnancy and lactation. Proteins are digested to supply essential amino acids, which make up the building blocks of the tissues of the body. It is important that the horse receives good quality protein in the diet, with adequate amounts of the amino acids lysine, methionine and cystine. Table 4.4 describes the appearance, nutritional value and feeding hints for some protein sources for horses. Fishmeal, cottonseed meal, sunflower meal and peanut meal can also be used as protein sources depending on their availability.

Table 4.4 Appearance, nutritional value and feeding hints for some protein sources.

Feed	Description	Nutritional value	Feeding hints
Linseed	Small, shiny, brown seeds	22% crude protein 18 MJ DE/kg 7% fibre 31% oil Low quality protein. Expensive. Largely replaced by soyabean meal	Palatable, good coat conditioner. Must be boiled to destroy poisons. During boiling absorbs a lot of water and becomes a jelly. Mild laxative properties
Soyabean (Fig. 4.5)	Raw beans contain toxin and must be heat treated. Can be either fat extracted (protein source) or full fat (energy and protein)	44% crude protein 13 MJ DE/kg 6% fibre 1% oil Full fat soya up to 20% fat	Very high quality protein for horses. Oil helps coat condition. Can be added to traditional hay and oat rations as sole protein source
Peas and beans	Peas are now more common than beans. Fed micronised or steam flaked. May be sold as mixed flakes with maize and barley	24% crude protein 13 MJ DE/kg 6% fibre 5% oil Good source of lysine	Palatable, often included in coarse mixes. Traditionally added to winter diet of horses
Milk powder		34% crude protein 15 MJ DE/kg 0% fibre 0.6% oil High in lysine	Palatable. Energy not available to weaned animals. Expensive

Compound feeds

Compound feeds are the modern way to feed the nutrients required by the horse. They are produced as either cubes or low or high energy coarse mixes (Figs 4.6 and 4.7). They have many advantages over

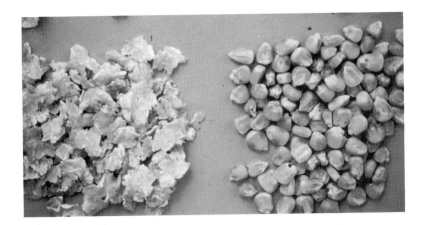

Fig. 4.4   Maize, whole and micronised. (Picture supplied courtesy of Dodson and Horrell Ltd.)

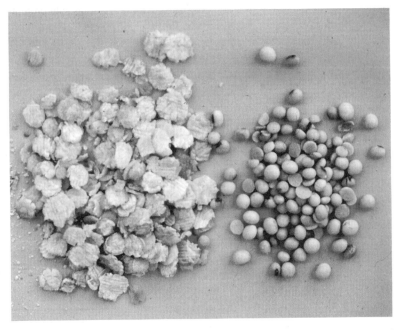

Fig. 4.5   Soyabean meal, whole, flaked and meal. (Picture supplied courtesy of Dodson and Horrell Ltd.)

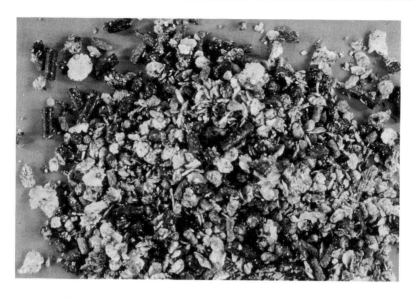

Fig. 4.6   A low energy mix. (Picture supplied courtesy of Dodson and Horrell Ltd.)

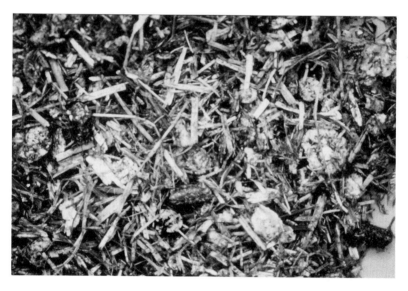

Fig. 4.7   A high energy mix. (Picture supplied courtesy of Dodson and Horrell Ltd.)

traditional straight feeds such as oats and barley. These advantages include:

- Convenience; the feeds contain everything the horse needs and do not require supplementation. This means you do not need to fill the feed room with lots of different types of feed.
- There are feeds for every type of horse, from foals to veterans.
- The feeds are of consistent quality and are produced under conditions of strict quality control. In addition, the manufacturer has to declare some of the nutrient values on a label attached to the bag so that you know what you are getting.
- Most products have a good shelf life and an expiry date so that you can ensure the food is fresh.
- They are virtually dust-free, making them suitable for feeding to horses with a dust allergy.
- They are highly palatable. Coarse mixes are specially designed to tempt fussy feeders and care must be taken not to overfeed them.

Some people distrust cubes, worried that you cannot tell good quality from poor quality ingredients. Most reputable feed manufacturers now list the raw materials contained in a cube on the bag or a label attached to the bag. If you are in doubt ring the manufacturer and seek advice from their nutritionist. Ingredients of cubes and coarse mixes include:

- Oats, barley, wheat, maize, peas, beans
- Soya, linseed
- Wheatfeed, oatfeed, nutritionally improved straw
- Alfa-beet
- Grassmeal, alfalfa, chaff
- Oil
- Vitamins and minerals
- Herbs
- Molasses.

Another criticism levelled at cubes is that horses find them boring to eat. It is probably more accurate to say that horse owners find them boring to feed; after all, horses eat grass all their lives and do not become bored with that. Undoubtedly some horses find the texture of cubes unappealing; these animals will often eat a coarse mix.

Look on the bag. Manufacturers will declare the:

- % Protein
- % Oil
- % Fibre
- % Ash
- Vitamins A, D and E (iu/kg)
- Copper (amount depends on manufacturer).

They may add further information such as the percentage of starch and the energy level of the feed. The ash is a measure of the non-energy part of the feed; thus low ash feeds are usually high in energy. Remember: although you may be able to look at a sample of oats and decide that they are clean and plump you cannot see the protein and energy in them and there will be nothing on the bag to help you. The bag that a cube comes out of has to state its feed value. Cubes and mixes can supply the demands of most types of horse or pony. Table 4.5 shows examples of the range of feeds available.

Table 4.5 Examples of the range of compound feeds available.

Maintenance feeds for various workloads	Protein (%)	Oil (%)	Fibre (%)	Digestible energy (MJ DE/kg)
Rest or light work				
Mix	8.5	2.2	15	9
Cubes	9	2	18	8.5
Light to medium work				
Mix	10	3.25	11	10
Cubes	10	3.25	15	9.5
Medium to hard work				
Mix	12	3.25	8	12
Cubes	11.5	3.25	12	11
Hard, fast work				
Mix	14	5	6	14
Cubes	14	4	9.5	13
Old age	11	4.5	11	11
Showing condition	12	4.25	9	12

Feeding compounds

Few horse owners feed compounds according to the manufacturer's guidelines; they add oats or barley to them, believing that horses find them 'boring'. Adding grain to the mix unbalances the compound and defeats one of the reasons for feeding a compound which is feeding a convenient, balanced ration in one bag. If the horse needs more energy than the present cube is supplying, then buy a higher energy, competition mix. On the other hand, if the horse is too 'fresh' (lively or overexuberant) or becoming fat on the present mix, change to a lower energy cube.

Chapter 5
Simple Ration Formulation

Most horse owners feel at a loss when confronted with the grand term 'ration formulation'. How are they supposed to do the calculations, working out megajoules per day and protein requirements? Rationing – in other words, deciding how much and what to feed your horse – can be made more simple. The result of these simple steps will be a basic ration which should provide enough evergy, protein and bulk for your horse. Depending on your horse's individual quirks you can then fine tune this ration to get one exactly right for your horse. Depending on the feeds you choose to feed they may or may not provide sufficient minerals and vitamins; this is where the nutritionist comes in.

There are many factors to consider when deciding on what and how much to feed a horse. These include:

- Height – large horses eat more than small ones.
- Breed/type – native breeds and cobs need less food than thoroughbreds.
- Age – young and old horses have special requirements.
- Condition – is the horse fat or thin?
- Amount of natural energy – some horses are naturally more energetic than others and may need fewer concentrates.
- Is the horse a good- or poor-doer? Unlike farm animals, horses have not been selected and bred for their ability to convert food efficiently. So we see a great difference in an individual horse's ability to utilise its food. Even within breeds some, just like us, are naturally lean or plump.
- How is the horse kept? Is it stabled or kept at grass?
- If the horse gets turned out, what amount and quality of grass is available?
- The time of year will affect the feed requirement.
- When were the horse's teeth last rasped?
- When was the horse last wormed?

- Does the horse have any allergies, e.g. to rolled barley or hay?
- If the horse is a brood mare, is she barren, in foal or has she got a foal at foot?
- What is the horse's temperament like? Can it tolerate concentrate feeds?
- How much work is the horse doing?

Remember that in order to thrive on its feed a horse must be regularly and effectively wormed and have its teeth checked twice a year and rasped if necessary.

Working out a ration

In the practical situation when a new horse arrives in the yard you have to decide what to put on the feed board immediately; there is no time to get out your calculator! All you have to do is follow four simple steps:

(1) Estimate the horse's bodyweight and condition score.
(2) Decide on the horse's appetite.
(3) Decide on the ratio of roughage to concentrates.
(4) Calculate the ration.

Bodyweight and condition score

The first thing to do is to decide how large the horse is and how much it weighs, as the amount a horse eats is proportional to its size or bodyweight. Most horses eat about 2–2.5% of their bodyweight per day. Many people find it tricky to estimate the bodyweight of their horse; it is a technique that requires much practice. It is important to have some idea of your horse's bodyweight so that it can be fed and wormed correctly. Horse owners (and vets) may underestimate a horse's weight. Many feed manufacturers base their feeding recommendations on the horse's weight and overestimating how much your horse weighs can lead to it being overfed and result in behavioural problems. Often the feed is blamed for being 'too heating' whereas a reduction of concentrates and an increase in hay may well solve the problem.

Bodyweight is proportional to the horse's girth diameter and the height and length of the body. This will be affected by the horse's type, build, breed and condition. Obviously using a weighbridge is the most accurate way to measure a horse's bodyweight, but not many of us have access to one. Alternatively a calculation relating girth and length can be used. However, rather than getting out your calculator, a simple method of estimating the horse's weight is to place a weightape around the horse's girth (Fig. 5.1), and use Table 5.1 to give an approximate guide to the relationship between height, girth and bodyweight. Weightapes may be only 85% accurate as they cannot take into account the horse's condition and type, but if you use one regularly it will help you monitor if your horse is becoming fatter or thinner.

Table 5.1   Relationship between height, girth and bodyweight.

Height		Girth		Bodyweight	
(hh)	(cm)	(cm)	(in)	(kg)	(lb)
11	111	135–145	53–57	200–260	440–572
12	122	140–150	55–59	230–290	506–638
13	132	150–160	59–63	290–350	638–770
14	142	160–170	63–67	350–420	770–924
15	152	170–185	67–73	420–520	924–1144
16	162	185–195	73–77	500–600	1100–1320
17	172	195–210	77–83	600–725	1320–1595

How much the horse weighs will also be affected by how much condition it is carrying. This will also affect how much you feed a horse – a thin horse will need more to eat than a fat horse. Once you have calculated the basic ration, you will need to alter it, taking into account the horse's condition. If you see a horse every day it can be more difficult to notice slight changes in condition. Perhaps it is only when a friend, who sees the horse less often, comments on the horse's increased (or decreased) waistline. Regular use of a weightape will help you keep track of whether the horse is losing or gaining weight, but it will not tell you if the horse is the right weight for the work it is doing. A show horse would look fat in a racing yard and a racehorse would look too lean in a showing yard. An objective way to assess a horse's condition is through a method called condition scoring. This involves looking at and feeling the horse to determine the amount and distribution of body fat, using a scoring

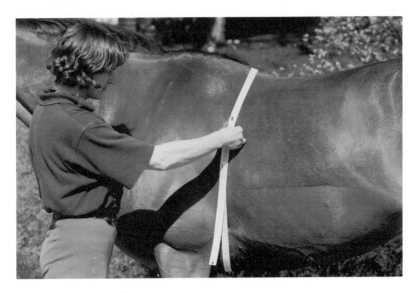

Fig. 5.1 Using a weightape.

system from 0 to 5, assessing the back ribs and over the quarters (Fig. 5.2).

To condition score a horse stand directly behind it and note the amount of flesh covering the pelvis and top of the quarters, the flanks and beneath the tail, assess the tautness of skin over the pelvis and compare your findings with the comments in Table 5.2. The backbone and ribs are scored by observing and feeling the horse from both sides.

Condition score	1	2	3	4	5
	Thin	Moderately thin	Moderately fleshy	Fat	Obese
Hind view					

Fig. 5.2 Condition scoring.

Table 5.2 Condition scoring.

Condition score	Quarters	Back and ribs	Neck and shoulders
0–extremely emaciated	Deep cavity under tail and either side of croup. Pelvis angular. No detectable fatty tissue between skin and bone	Processes of vertebrae sharp to touch. Skin drawn tightly over ribs	'Ewe-neck' (neck shaped like a sheep's neck), very narrow, individual bone structure visible. Bone structure of shoulder visible. No fatty tissue
1–thin	Pelvis and croup well defined, no fatty tissue, but skin supple. Poverty lines (deep lines running down hindquarters either side of tail) visible and deep depression under tail	Ribs and backbone clearly defined, but skin slack over bones	'Ewe-neck', narrow, flat muscle covering. Shoulder accentuated, some fat
2–moderately thin	Croup well defined, but some fatty tissue under skin. Pelvis easily felt, slight depression under tail. Not obviously thin	Backbone just covered by fatty tissue, individual processes not visible, but easily felt on pressure. Ribs just visible	Narrow but firm. Shoulder not obviously thin
3–moderately fleshy	Whole pelvic region rounded, not angular and no 'gutter' (depression) along croup. Skin smooth and supple, pelvis easily felt	Backbone and ribs well covered, but easily felt on pressure	Neck blends smoothly into body. No crest except for stallions. Layer of fat over shoulder

Contd

Table 5.2 contd

Condition score	Quarters	Back and ribs	Neck and shoulders
4–fat	Pelvis buried in fatty tissue and only felt on firm pressure. 'Gutter' over croup	Backbone and ribs well covered and only felt on firm pressure. 'Gutter' along backbone	Wide and firm with folds of fatty tissue, slight crest even in mares. Fat buildup behind shoulder
5–obese	Pelvis buried in firm, fatty tissue and cannot be felt. Clear, deep 'gutter' over croup to base of dock. Skin stretched	Back looks flat with deep 'gutter' along backbone. Ribs buried and cannot be felt	Very wide and firm, marked crest, even in mares. Shoulder bulging fat

Finally the neck is scored by standing by the horse's shoulder and noting the shape and feel of the neck just in front of the withers.

A horse with a condition score of 0 is starving, with sharp and prominent croup and hip bones, cut up behind (i.e. if you lift the tail the inner thigh is very lean) and with a prominent ribcage. A thin horse would have a condition score of 1; the bones are still prominent but there is more muscle definition (Fig. 5.3). Horses with a score of 2 are approaching normal; the hip bones and vertebrae of the back are defined but not prominent as would be expected in fit horses, such as hunters and eventers (Fig. 5.4). Those with a score of 3 are getting fat and the bones become more difficult to feel, as one would expect with a horse in show condition (Fig. 5.5). Scores 4 and 5 indicate obesity, with large masses of fat on the neck, quarters and back (Figs 5.6 and 5.7). The ribs can only be felt on pressure.

Ideal condition score

Hard working horses such as endurance horses and eventers are usually kept in lower body condition than dressage horses and show horses. Table 5.3 shows the optimum condition score for different types of horses. If a horse is too fat or too thin then it may be necessary to adjust both the diet and the work regime to correct the situation.

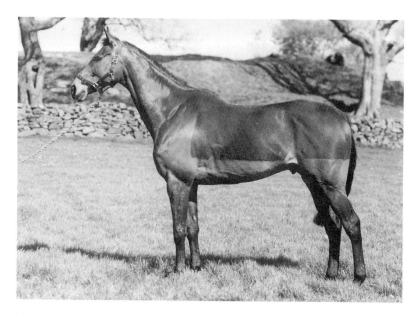

(a)

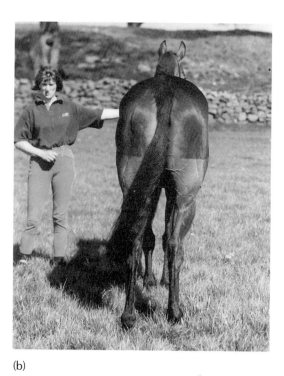

(b)

Fig. 5.3   A lean, unfit horse with a condition score between 1 and 2, (a) side view, (b) hind view.

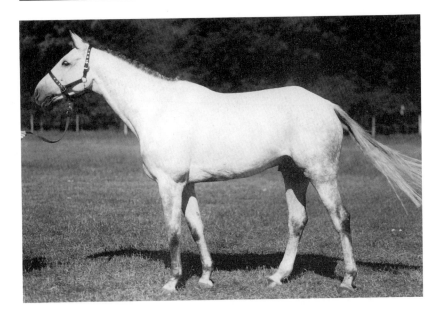

(a)

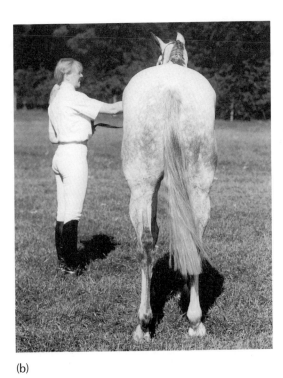

(b)

Fig. 5.4   A lean three-day event horse, condition score 2, (a) side view, (b) hind view.

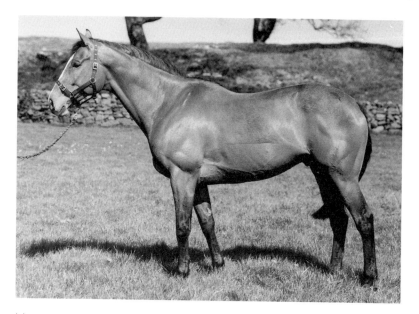

(a)

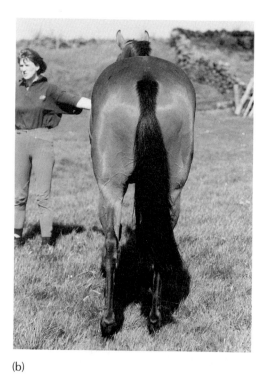

(b)

Fig. 5.5   A rounded, fit horse, condition score between 2 and 3, (a) side view, (b) hind view.

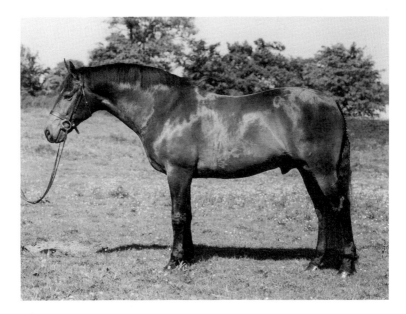

(a)

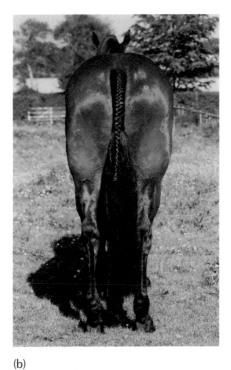

(b)

Fig. 5.6   A fat horse, condition score 4, (a) side view, (b) hind view.

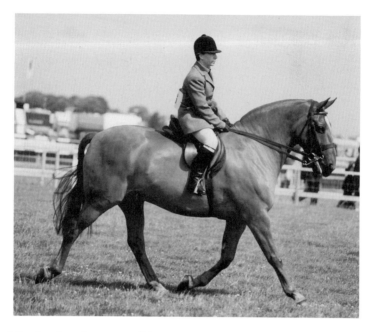

Fig. 5.7   An obese horse, condition score 5.

Table 5.3   Optimum condition score for different types of horses.

Type of horse	Condition score (0–thin, 5–obese)
Dressage	3
Endurance	2–3
Eventer	2–3
Racehorses	2–3
Hunter	3
Barren mare	2–3
Polo pony	3
Pregnant mare	3–4
Show jumper	3
Show horse	4
Ponies on spring grass	Not more than 4

Condition scoring is also useful if you are worried about fat ponies suffering from laminitis. Once a week make a note of the pony's condition score and the size of its crest (Fig. 5.8). In addition, make sure that its toes never get too long and check the rate of growth of the

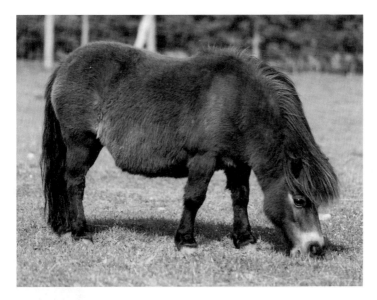

Fig. 5.8   A cresty pony which could be prone to laminitis.

grass at least twice a week. If the pony is getting obese and the grass is growing quickly the pony must have its grazing restricted and, if possible, its exercise increased.

Appetite

Table 5.4 shows the amounts of dry food a horse needs to eat every day in order to maintain condition and bodyweight. This will vary according to the horse's bodyweight and the amount of work it is doing. Thus, a resting, 16-hh (162-cm) horse weighing 500 kg (1100 lb) needs only eat 7.5 kg (16.5 lb) dry weight of food a day to maintain its bodyweight. Most horses will happily eat 2.5% of their bodyweight as dry matter a day, which is why resting horses tend to put on weight. The same horse in moderate work will eat 12.5 kg (27.5 lb) feed every day, i.e.

$$\frac{500 \times 2.5}{100} = 12.5 \text{ kg}$$

As the horse's workload increases so does the amount of food that it needs to eat, so this horse in intense work would eat up to 15 kg (33 lb)

Table 5.4 Relationship between bodyweight (given in kg and lb), work level and appetite, showing amount of dry food a horse needs daily to maintain condition and bodyweight.

Work level and appetite	200 kg 440 lb	400 kg 900 lb	450 kg 1000 lb	500 kg 1100 lb	550 kg 1200 lb	600 kg 1320 lb
Resting 1.5% bodyweight	3 kg 6.5 lb	6 kg 13 lb	7 kg 15 lb	7.5 kg 16.5 lb	8 kg 17 lb	9 kg 20 lb
Light work 2% bodyweight	4 kg 9 lb	8 kg 17 lb	9 kg 20 lb	10 kg 22 lb	11 kg 24 lb	12 kg 26.5 lb
Moderate work 2.5% bodyweight	5 kg 11 lb	10 kg 22 lb	11.5 kg 25 lb	12.5 kg 27.5 lb	13.5 kg 30 lb	14.5 kg 32 lb
Intense work 2.5–3% bodyweight	6 kg 13 lb	12 kg 26.5 lb	13.5 kg 30 lb	15 kg 33 lb	16.5 kg 36 lb	18 kg 40 lb

dry food every day to help to fuel the workload. Unfortunately some horses lose their appetite when worked hard (see 'Poor appetite after work', Chapter 12).

Ratio of roughage to concentrates

A rule of thumb that has been used for many years to help decide what to ration horses has been a simple table, relating the intensity of the horse's work to the ratio of roughage to concentrates fed, as shown in Table 5.5. The horse in light work will need more hay and less energy feed, while the horse in hard work will need less hay and a greater proportion of high energy, hard feed. The ration should be based on roughage using Table 5.5; the energy shortfall can then be made up by the concentrate ration. The final weight of the daily feed may be less than shown in Table 5.4 if high energy feeds like oil are used. Horses in hard work may not be able to eat 3% of their bodyweight, especially if they are fussy eaters, so their appetite should be calculated using 2.5% bodyweight and energy-rich foods used to provide the required energy levels.

Table 5.5 A guide to the ratio of roughage to concentrates.

Work level	% Roughage	% Concentrate
Resting	90–100	0–10
Light	75–80	20–25
Moderate	65–70	30–35
Hard	55–65	35–45
Intense	40–50	50–60

It is recommended that roughage should make up at least 50% of the ration; however, the greater the physical activity, the less bulk the horse is likely to consume. The concentrate level may be increased by 10% during periods of hard training and competition to compensate for this. When feeding this amount of concentrates care must be taken to reduce the feed before and during rest days.

Horse owners often overestimate the amount of work that their horses are doing. Just because you get off the horse feeling exhausted this does not mean that the horse has worked equally hard; horses are expert at making us work while doing very little themselves! Remember that you must take into consideration the horse's overall workload, so that even if you go for long rides at the weekend, if the horse does nothing during the week overall its workload is very light.

- Light work – hacking and light competition.
- Moderate work – regular competition, e.g. one-day horse trials.
- Hard work – hunting, advanced competition, e.g. three-day eventing.
- Intense work – racing.

Table 5.6 shows how the ration would vary depending on the horse's workload.

The ration

For our example ration let us take a 16-hh (162-cm) horse in hard work:

- The horse weighs 500 kg (1100 lb) (Table 5.1).

Table 5.6 Rations for varying work levels.

Work level	Hay	Concentrate	Comment
Resting	10–12 kg 22–26.5 lb	1–2 kg 2–4 lb	Amount depends on weather, amount of grass, etc.
Light	9–10 kg 20–22 lb	2.5–3 kg 5.5–6.5 lb	Low energy cubes
Moderate	8–9 kg 17–20 lb	4–4.5 kg 9–10 lb	Medium energy cubes
Hard	6.5–8 kg 14–17 lb	4.5–5.5 kg 10–12 lb	High energy feed
Intense	5–6 kg 11–13 lb	6–7.5 kg 13–16.5 lb	Racehorse mix or cubes/naked oats

- It will have an appetite of 12.5 kg (27.5 lb) (Table 5.4).
- It will be fed 40% concentrates and 60% roughage (Table 5.5).

This results in a ration of 5 kg (11 lb) concentrates and 7.5 kg (16.5 lb) roughage. The next step is to decide what concentrates to feed, depending on the horse's individual requirements and your personal preference.

Monitoring condition

Once a ration has been made up for a horse and written on the feed board it is vital to monitor that horse's reaction to the new ration. Ask yourself some questions:

- Does the horse eat up? If the horse is leaving food it may be that you have overestimated its appetite, the food is not palatable or the horse is feeling off-colour.
- Are the horse's temperament and performance affected?
- Is the horse gaining, losing or maintaining condition?

A diet too high in energy may make the horse 'hot' (overexuberant) and it will grow fatter, while too little energy will result in loss of condition and possibly a lethargic temperament. Some horses are naturally 'hot' no matter how little they are fed and it must be remembered that training, fitness and discipline will also affect temperament.

Condition of the skin and coat

A good diet should not just keep the horse in good condition; the horse should also look well in itself (Fig. 5.9). The coat should be glossy and feel smooth and silky; the skin should be loose and pliable, and when picked up in a pinch and released should return smoothly and easily to its former position. Any delay indicates either a degree of dehydration or a lack of subcutaneous fat.

Condition of the teeth

A tooth problem can make a horse difficult to ride and cause it to lose condition. Do not overlook this simple management check. Teeth must be looked at and rasped regularly – at least twice a year, and as often as every 6 weeks if the horse has a problem.

Condition of the hooves

Dry, flaky and brittle hooves can be an indication that the horse's diet is not balanced, although the effect of shoeing and environment cannot be ignored. If the horse is receiving a good quality diet and looks well in all other respects, it may be suffering from a specific shortage of hoof-forming elements. The substances involved in building up and maintaining healthy hoof horn include biotin, sulphur, zinc, lysine and methionine and supplements containing these minerals, vitamins and amino acids.

Practical adjustments to the ration

Once you have calculated the ration your horse needs and decided which type of concentrates you are going to feed you need to assess your horse's individual reaction to that diet.

- If the horse consistently leaves feed you may have overestimated its appetite. Reduce the hay by 10–20%. Increase the concentrates by 5–10% to maintain the energy content of the ration. This reduces the overall amount the horse receives, but maintains the nutrient intake.

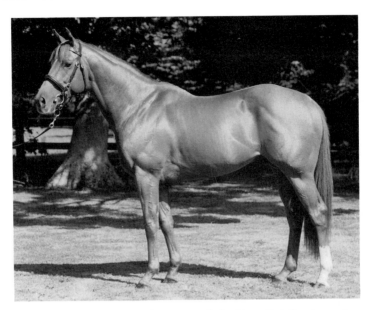

Fig. 5.9 A horse in superb condition, rounded with well defined muscle and a gleaming coat.

- If the horse is eating everything and still appears to be hungry you may have underestimated its appetite. In this case increase the hay by 10% and reduce the concentrate feed by 5%. The extra bulk will keep the horse occupied, but it will not get fatter as its concentrate ration has been cut. Table 5.7 shows how the ration can be adjusted to cater for individual horses depending on their appetites by altering the relative amount of hay and concentrate in the feed.

- On rest days the concentrate ration should be at least halved, preferably starting the evening before. The full ration should be resumed gradually over 2 days after work starts, as follows:

Evening feed before rest day	Half nomal concentrate feed	Extra hay
Rest day	Half normal concentrate feed	Extra hay
Next work day	Three-quarters normal concentrate feed	Extra hay
Next day	Full feed	Normal hay ration

Table 5.7 Adjusting the ration to cater for individual horse appetites.

Adjustment to concentrate	Concentrate (kg)	(lb)	Adjustment to hay	Hay (kg)	(lb)	Total (kg)	(lb)
Original ration	5	11	—	7.5	16.5	12.5	27.5
Poor appetite Increase by 5%	5.25	11.5	Decrease by 10%	6.75	15	12	26.5
OR Increase by 10%	5.5	12	Decrease by 20%	6	13	11.5	25
Hungry horse Decrease by 5%	4.75	10.5	Increase by 10%	8.25	18	13	28.5
OR Decrease by 10%	4.5	10	Increase by 20%	9	20	13.5	30

- If a horse becomes overexuberant on the concentrate ration either change to a lower energy feed or substitute some oil; 100 ml (0.2 pt) oil is equivalent in energy terms to about 0.25 kg (0.5 lb) oats.
- The horse's bodyweight and condition score should be monitored to make sure that the horse is maintaining its bodyweight. Performance and temperament should also be noted.

Remember, each horse is an individual and should be treated as such. Poor-doers will need more feed while good-doers will need less if they are not to put on too much condition.

Chapter 6
Supplements

Who needs them?

Most of us feel guilty if we do not feed an expensive supplement, perhaps hoping it will make the horse perform just that little bit better, but do we really need to? The horse owner is swamped by products claiming to help our horses, from making them calmer, through reducing digestive upsets to helping them grow better feet. However, a supplement is not a recipe for success – it can only work if it corrects an imbalance or deficiency in the horse's diet or the horse has a specific requirement for a substance.

If a horse is in light to moderate work and is being fed a reputable compound feed at the manufacturer's recommended rate, receiving good quality hay and has access to grass, it should require nothing extra except some salt. Horses likely to require a supplement are stabled performance horses, growing youngsters, brood mares in late pregnancy and early lactation, old horses and those receiving poor quality hay, especially in winter. A traditional mixture of oats and hay is deficient in many micronutrients and horses that are not getting a compound feed will need a supplement.

What are they?

Supplements are substances added to the horse's diet to balance it by filling in deficiencies of certain nutrients, most often minerals, vitamins and amino acids. Do not confuse them with additives, which are substances added to an already balanced ration, for example probiotics and enzymes; these may have an indirect effect on the horse's health, but they are not fed for their nutritional value. Vitamins and minerals cannot be considered on their own. There are complicated interactions between them and other nutrients. For example, the form of mineral can affect its availability to the horse as well as how it will interact with other nutrients, for instance there is a relationship between selenium and vitamin E.

Supplements can vary in their complexity; one of the most simple supplements fed to horses is salt, while at the other end of the scale there are broad-spectrum supplements containing many nutrients. Broad-spectrum supplements are formulated on the basis of the average horse being fed an average ration, making up for likely deficiencies; some simple supplements cater for specific problems, e.g. biotin for hoof growth.

Minerals

Minerals can be classified as major minerals, electrolytes and trace elements. Fourteen are needed for healthy skeletal development, body function and metabolism in the horse. The need for a strong skeleton, efficient metabolism and tissue growth and repair increases the need for a balanced and adequate supply of minerals in the diet of the performance horse and the breeding and growing horse. Soil deficiencies, natural imbalances and the poor availability of certain minerals mean that the stabled horse, in particular, is unlikely to receive sufficient amounts from diets based on cereal grains and hay. A balanced mineral supplement or the provision of a specially formulated compound feed is essential for the performance horse and the breeding and growing horse.

Table 6.1 shows the minerals required by the horse on a daily basis.

Major minerals

Calcium and phosphorus

Calcium and phosphorus, along with vitamin D, are needed for bone development and strength. The amount needed depends on the horse's age, diet and workload, but should fall within a ratio of 2 calcium to 1 phosphorus. As there is more phosphorus than calcium in cereals, horses on high grain rations are likely to be deficient in calcium. Calcium can be supplied by adding ground limestone to the diet, while calcium and phosphorus are supplied by dicalcium phosphate.

Table 6.1 Mineral requirements of horses.

Minerals	Per kg of diet	Per day for 16–hh (500-kg) (1100-lb)
Calcium (g)		45*
Phosphorus (g)		30*
Sodium (g)	3.5	44
Potassium (g)	4	50
Magnesium (g)	0.9	11
Iron (mg)	150	1900
Copper (mg)	20	250
Cobalt (mg)	0.2	2.5
Manganese (mg)	50	625
Zinc (mg)	60	750
Selenium (mg)	0.2	2.5
Iodine (mg)	0.15	1.9
Sulphur (g)	1.5	19

* Amount depends on diet, age, workload, etc. These figures are average requirements of an adult horse in work.

On a hay and cereal diet you will need to add 25–30 g (approximately 1 oz) limestone flour per day. Most broad-spectrum supplements will contain some calcium and phosphorus, but probably not enough to balance the ration. The manufacturer does not know what you are going to feed, and the calcium and phosphorus requirements will vary depending on the horse's diet, age and reproductive status. If you are in any doubt, ring the manufacturer and ask for advice.

Electrolytes

Sodium, potassium, magnesium and chloride

Sodium, potassium and chloride are involved in nerve and muscle function and the fluid balance of the horse's body. Magnesium is interrelated to calcium and phosphorus in bone development. The amount of electrolytes a horse needs depends on its workload, the temperature and humidity, i.e. how much the horse sweats in training and in competition. A deficiency of these electrolytes results in dehydration and poor performance. Other factors such as sudden stress or dietary changes, e.g. a flush of spring grass, can increase the horse's need for magnesium. Magnesium loss has been associated with temperament problems and misbehaviour.

Whatever diet you are feeding you will need to add salt (sodium chloride). Salt can be added to the feed or offered as a salt lick in the manger or in a holder on the wall (Fig. 6.1). A salt lick in the manger can help stop the horse bolting its feed by slowing the horse down, but there is no guarantee that the horse will receive enough salt. On the other hand, it may devour the lick, drink to compensate and have a very wet bed. Many horses will not use a salt lick on the wall and the holder is a projection that the horse may injure itself on. Salt that is added to the feed can be monitored and you can be sure the horse eats it. The performance horse should have at least 40 g (1–2 tablespoons) common salt per day added to its feed. Horses and ponies that are not working so hard could rely on a salt lick either in their manger or out in the field. Grazing horses that eat soil and bark may be seeking salt and should be offered a salt lick in the field (Fig. 6.2).

Trace elements

Iron, copper and cobalt

Iron, copper and cobalt are involved in red blood cell production and are important in the diet of the performance horse. Copper is also important in the growth and development of young horses. Traditional diets tend to be low in copper and certain areas of the country are deficient in it; specialised supplements are available to counteract this. A supplement designed to help the anaemic horse is likely to contain these trace elements.

Manganese

Manganese is important to maintain metabolism and musculo-skeletal function. However, it is unlikely to be deficient in the horse.

Zinc

Zinc is involved in the health of the skin and cartilage and hoof formation. While a deficiency is not likely, zinc is often included in supplements designed to enhance skin and coat condition and to improve hoof growth.

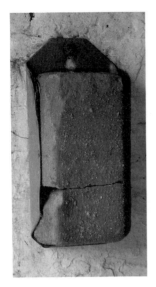

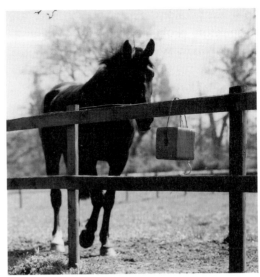

Fig. 6.1 Salt lick on a stable wall.

Fig. 6.2 Salt lick in the field.

Selenium

Selenium works with vitamin E to protect the muscles from damage during exercise. Selenium is marginally deficient in many areas of the UK; however, it must also be remembered that excess selenium is highly poisonous. Selenium and vitamin E are often used in supplements which attempt to prevent 'tying-up' (azoturia) in performance horses.

Iodine

Iodine is associated with the thyroid gland which controls the body's metabolic rate. Deficiency may occur, while oversupplementation with seaweed-based supplements may lead to an iodine excess.

Sulphur

Sulphur is contained in the amino acids methionine and cystine, so a horse that is receiving adequate high quality protein should not have a problem. While a clinical deficiency is not recognised, there are several supplements that contain organic sulphur. These are said to help skin and hoof condition, to act as an anti-inflammatory and to help with respiratory problems. Much of the information is anecdotal, but many horse owners swear by it!

Molybdenum

Molybdenum deficiency is not known in the horse, but excess amounts may increase the horse's requirement for copper.

Fluorine

Fluorine is important in bone and teeth development. Deficiency is not a problem in horses and there are no proven benefits of supplementation.

Chromium

Chromium is an essential trace element which can be used to reduce anxiety. In performance horses it is also said to maximise energy utilisation and recovery after exercise.

Vitamins

Compared with other nutrients, vitamins are only required in very small amounts. Sixteen vitamins are required for healthy body function in the horse. The horse's requirement for vitamins will depend on its age, growth rate, reproductive status and workload. Extra amounts of vitamins are needed by foals, brood mares and performance horses. Many of the feeds commonly fed to horses are deficient in or have unbalanced levels of vitamins; this is due to the processes of harvesting, treatment and storage that the feedstuffs undergo.

Table 6.2 shows the vitamins required by the horse on a daily basis.

Fat-soluble vitamins

Vitamin A (retinol)

Vitamin A helps ensure red blood cell production, tendon strength, skin condition and performance. The precursor of vitamin A, carotene,

Table 6.2 Vitamin requirements of horses.

Vitamin	Total requirement	Per day
Vitamin A	12 000 iu/kg	Up to 50 000 iu for performance horses
Vitamin D_3	1200 iu/kg	Up to 6000 iu for performance horses. Adequate calcium and phosphorus must be present in diet
Vitamin E	Up to 200 iu/kg	Up to 1800 iu for performance horses. 100 iu extra vitamin E should be supplied for every 100 ml oil in ration
Vitamin K	Unknown	Up to 20 mg in feed
Vitamin B_1 (thiamine)	15 mg/kg	50–100 mg. 3000 mg has been said to reduce nervous behaviour
Vitamin B_2 (riboflavin)	15 mg/kg	Up to 50 mg
Vitamin B_3 (niacin)	25 mg/kg	Up to 400 mg
Vitamin B_5 (pantothenic acid)	15 mg/kg	Up to 100 mg
Vitamin B_6 (pyridoxine)	10 mg/kg	Up to 50 mg
Vitamin B_{12}	250 µg/kg	Deficiency not common
Folic acid	10 mg/kg	Up to 15 mg
Biotin	0.2 mg/kg	15 mg aids hoof strength and growth
Choline	200 mg/kg	Up to 600 mg
Vitamin C	250 mg/kg	450 mg is needed to increase blood levels

is rapidly destroyed in feedstuffs during processing and storage which means that stabled horses in winter are likely to need a supplement. Green pasture contains adequate amounts of carotene to supply grazing horses with vitamin A.

Vitamin D₃ (cholecalciferol)

Vitamin D_3 is involved with calcium and phosphorus in bone formation. It is synthesised by the action of sunlight on the horse's skin, and horses need up to 20 minutes of bright sunshine daily to provide enough vitamin D from the skin. Stabled horses in winter and performance horses with limited access to grass are likely to need a supplement.

Vitamin E (alpha-tocopherol)

Vitamin E is closely involved with selenium in muscle function. Vitamin and selenium supplements may aid muscle strength and reduce the incidence of 'tying-up' (azoturia). Growing horses and performance horses have a high requirement for vitamin E; high fat diets also increase the horse's vitamin E requirement. These horses will need supplementary vitamin E.

Vitamin K (menadione)

Vitamin K is produced by the micro-organisms in the hind gut and is involved in blood clotting. Although a deficiency is unlikely, supplementation may be beneficial prior to major surgery.

Water-soluble vitamins

Vitamin B complex is a group of water-soluble vitamins. All the B vitamins are involved in the metabolism of the body which means that performance horses have a high B vitamin requirement and that a deficiency of B vitamins shows itself as poor or reduced performance. These vitamins are synthesised by the micro-organisms in the intestine so that the grazing horse in moderate work is unlikely to have a problem. However, the performance horse with limited access to grass and a high concentrate, low fibre diet is likely to need supplementation. Stress also reduces the gut synthesis of these vitamins. Supplementation will help the horse use a high energy diet more effectively, maintain appetite, maintain the red blood cell level and support performance.

Vitamin B₁ (thiamine)

Horses that get bracken poisoning are suffering from vitamin B_1 deficiency; they show signs of poor appetite, loss of condition and nervousness. These signs can usually be reversed by supplementing the diet with B_1 and making sure the horse cannot eat bracken. High levels of B_1 are sometimes fed to help maintain calmness and reduce nervous behaviour.

Vitamin B₂ (riboflavin), B₃ (niacin) and B₅ (pantothenic acid)

Vitamins B_2, B_7 and B_5 are involved in general body metabolism and are needed for performance. They are all synthesised in the gut, but production is reduced when the horse is under stress.

Biotin

Biotin is most well known for its role in hoof quality. Biotin and calcium are both needed for hoof bonding; 15 mg biotin daily aids hoof strength and growth.

Vitamin B₆ (pyridoxine), B₁₂ (cobalamine) and Folic acid

Vitamins B_6, B_{12} and folic acid are involved in red blood cell production. They are often included in supplements designed to help horses recovering from anaemia.

Choline

Choline is involved in the metabolism of fats. There is unlikely to be a deficiency because it can be synthesised in the liver from the amino acid methionine.

Vitamin C (ascorbic acid)

Unlike humans, the horse is able to make its own vitamin C and is very unlikely to be deficient. High levels of vitamin C have been fed to racehorses to try to prevent exercise-induced pulmonary haemorrhage (bleeding) and to reduce stress; however, there is no proof that it is effective.

What to look for in a supplement

A stabled horse is likely to require vitamins A, D_3 and E, plus folic acid. A selection of B vitamins may be necessary for performance horses receiving a high level of concentrates and with limited access to grass. Of all the trace elements, inadequate intakes of copper, selenium, manganese, iodine and zinc are most frequently detected and should be included in a supplement. Unless you are feeding a high quality protein look out for lysine and methionine in your supplement.

Supplements for the respiratory system

Keeping a horse free of respiratory problems is essential to performance and horse owners have been using garlic for a long time for this reason. Some additives consist of a syrup given to the horse before exercise; these often contain menthol and act in a similar way to the vapour rub or inhaler that you would use if you had a cold. Other supplements aim to maintain the body's natural defences against a dusty environment and to maintain the lung tissue. Methyl sulphonyl methane (MSM) and vitamins C and K may be included.

Guidelines for feeding supplements

- Make sure you read the manufacturer's instructions before using the supplement. Use the measure provided and replace the lid tightly after use.
- Store in a cool, dry place and avoid exposure to strong sunlight.
- Supplements should not be mixed or overdosed without advice from a vet or nutritionist.
- Make sure that you buy an appropriate amount so that you can use it all before its sell-by date.
- Remember that compound feeds are already supplemented; if you are feeding your horse the amount of cubes recommended by the manufacturers, you should not need another supplement.
- Few horses are receiving the maximum amount recommended by the feed manufacturer. Ring the manufacturer up and find out the minimum amount of mix or cube that will supply the

minerals and vitamins your horse needs. If you are not feeding that much you will need to add a certain amount of supplement to make up the balance.

- In theory, the supplement should be fed in each feed – not just the evening feed, as most often happens, as horses should not experience sudden changes to their diet. Split the supplement between all the feeds.
- If you are feeding a hot feed like a mash, wait for it to cool down before adding the supplement, otherwise nutrients may be denatured. If you feed a bran mash be sure to add some extra calcium to compensate for the low calcium level in bran.
- Like any new feed, introduce supplements gradually, taking about a week to build up to the full dose.
- Mix the supplement thoroughly into the feed.

Remember, unless the horse has a specific problem, a supplement is only necessary if:

- The horse is being fed poor quality feedstuffs
- High performance is required
- The horse is under stress, such as old age, illness or growth.

Chapter 7
Worms, Worming and Wormers

The horse is host to a large variety of internal parasites, most of which are the larval and adult stages of gastrointestinal 'worms'. Horses are susceptible to different types of worms at different stages in their life (Table 7.1). Of primary importance in the young foal are ascarids and threadworms, while the redworms are by far the most serious worm infections in older horses. Worm control is a vital aspect of any horse management programme and can be made more effective by an understanding of the life cycles of these parasites and a knowledge of the drugs available for their control.

Table 7.1 Types of worm affecting horses at different ages.

Foal	Threadworm
	Ascarid
Up to 3 years	Ascarid
	Large redworm
	Small redworm
	Bots
	Tapeworm
	Pinworm
Adult	Large redworm
	Small redworm
	Bots
	Tapeworm
	Pinworm

Ascarids (*Parascaris equorum*)

Ascarids are large round worms, which may be 30 cm (12 in) long and as thick as a pencil. An adult, egg-laying female living in the small intestine can lay from 200 000 to 1 million eggs per day; the eggs have a tough, sticky, outer coat which makes them very resistant to disinfectants and the environment, allowing them to survive for up to 3 years outside the horse. Infective larvae develop inside the egg and, when eaten by the foal, the larvae hatch in the foal's gut and burrow through the gut wall and migrate via the bloodstream to the liver and lungs. The larvae are coughed up, swallowed and undergo their final development to become egg-laying adults inside the small intestine. It takes 8–12 weeks from infection (the foal eating the eggs) for the larvae to mature and for eggs to start being passed out in the foal's droppings and thus infecting the pasture. From the eggs being passed out of the foal in the dung to the development of infective larvae takes about 30 days under optimal conditions. Foals should be wormed from 6 weeks of age – well before the ascarids reach full size and start egg laying. The life cycle is shown in Fig. 7.1.

A foal may have up to 1000 adult ascarids in its gut, causing the foal to have a dull coat, pot-belly, loss of condition and slow growth. The worms will cause inflammation of the lining of the gut and in severe cases may actually block the small intestine, causing rupture, peritonitis and death. The migrating larvae can cause coughing and a nasal discharge. Very heavy contamination can occur on paddocks grazed every year by mares and foals; mares must be wormed regularly during pregnancy, and ideally foals would only be turned out onto pasture

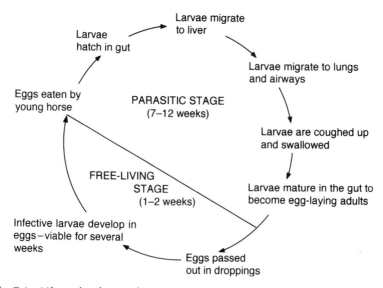

Fig. 7.1   Life cycle of ascarid.

that had not been grazed by horses in the previous 12 months. After the age of two, horses develop resistance to ascarids and these worms do not cause problems in older horses.

Threadworms (*Strongyloides westeri*)

Threadworms are a parasite of foals which can be passed from the mare via her milk or can enter the foal by penetrating the foal's skin. The adults live in the small intestine and are very small and generally well tolerated; however, heavy infection can cause scouring in foals of 2–4 weeks old which may coincide with the mare's foaling heat (the first time the mare comes into season after foaling). Foals can be treated for threadworm from 7 days old, but regular worming of the mare will help reduce the incidence and severity of threadworm infection. Infection is rarely seen in youngstock more than 6 months old. Threadworms are also roundworms and they are difficult to control, requiring high dosage or the use of ivermectin.

Large redworms (*Strongylus vulgaris*)

The large redworm was once the most important parasite affecting the horse because the migrating larval stages cause damage to the lining of arteries, particularly those supplying the gut. In severe cases the blood supply to the gut can be blocked by a clot, causing colic and even death. Modern worming programmes have successfully reduced the problem. Large redworms are roundworms, 2–8 cm long and coloured red from the blood that they suck. Eggs are laid by the adult worm in the large intestine of the horse and passed out in the droppings. The eggs can remain viable on the paddock until late May or early June of the following year. The eggs develop on the grass and become infective third stage (L3) larvae; the speed of this development depends upon the climate and takes about 10 days in warm, moist conditions. The L3 larvae are eaten by the grazing horse and pass into the intestines.

Large redworms migrate extensively through the body; about 8 days after infection the L3 larvae become so-called L4 larvae and migrate to the anterior mesenteric artery which is responsible for supplying most of the gut with blood. This migration damages the artery walls and causes blood clots; these clots may block smaller blood vessels and thus disrupt the blood supply to the gut, causing colic; indeed, redworms are thought to be the most common cause of recurrent bouts of spasmodic colic. Eventually the mature larvae return to the wall of the large intestine before emerging into the gut where they become egg-laying adults 5–9 months after infection. The life cycle is shown in Fig. 7.2.

This prolonged migration may lead to 'false negative' faecal worm egg counts; there may be no adult egg-laying worms in the gut and thus a negative worm egg count will be recorded, even though the tissues may contain many larvae which are causing extensive damage and will eventually become adults in the gut. Most wormers will effectively remove the adult stages, but high levels of fenbendazole or ivermectin are necessary to remove the migrating stages.

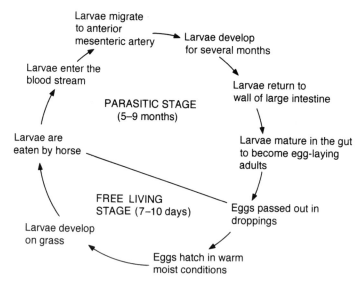

Fig. 7.2   Life cycle of large redworm.

Small redworms

There are 40 different species of small redworm (a roundworm). In recent years they have become the most important parasite of horses; this is due to their life cycle (Fig. 7.3) and the development of resistance to the benzimidazole group of wormers. The larvae are picked up by the grazing horse and in the spring and the summer they become egg-

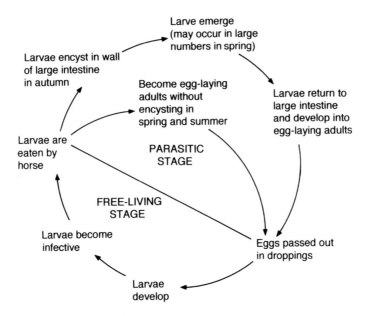

Fig. 7.3   Life cycle of small redworm.

laying adults 4–8 weeks after ingestion. This short life cycle means that several generations of larvae will be passed out in one grazing season; consequently pasture contamination can become very heavy indeed, leading to high worm burdens in the horse.

In the autumn, the small redworms burrow into the wall of the gut and are called encysted larvae. These larvae can remain dormant for many months; few wormers are active against them, while some are effective in high doses. This means that it is very important to worm regularly throughout the year to keep the population of developing larvae at low levels, so that in the autumn as few larvae as possible become encysted. In the late winter or spring, the larvae are triggered to continue their development and emerge into the gut. The high risk period is December to May. Large numbers entering the gut may cause:

- Weight loss
- Diarrhoea
- Sluggish behaviour
- Loss of appetite
- Colic
- Filled legs

- Fever
- Dehydration
- Possibly death.

In the past the high risk times for infection by small redworm were the spring and summer. The recent mild winters, hot, dry summers and warm, wet autumns have led to high levels of infective larvae on pasture all year round, even in January. This means that worming is important all year round in horses with access to pasture, not just in the grazing season. Redworms can affect horses of all ages. Foals less than 6 weeks old will not harbour any egg-laying adults, but the larval stages will start to cause damage soon after being eaten.

Controlling redworm infection

- Regular worming every 4–10 weeks between March and September will control the number of egg-laying adults and thus the number of infective larvae on the grass. This in turn means fewer larvae will become encysted.
- At present the only way to remove encysted larvae is to use fenbendazole for 5 consecutive days. While this may not be desirable as it will encourage resistant strains of worms, it is probably the best way to treat a new horse whose worming history is unknown.
- The manufacturers recommend a 5-day course in early November to remove the larvae picked up in the summer and again in February to remove the larvae which have encysted over the winter from winter grazing.
- Regular testing of the droppings for worm eggs will tell you if the worm population has become resistant to the benzimidazole wormers, in which case ivermectin or pyrantel should be used.
- Wormers should be rotated on an annual basis to avoid resistance developing.

Pinworms or seatworms (*Oxyuris equi*)

The pinworm is a white, round worm, 1–10 cm long and 1 mm diameter. It is killed by routine doses of wormer and is not usually a problem; the adults live in the large intestine, the female lays her eggs on the skin surrounding the anus, which causes intense itching. Larvae develop within 4 days; they then fall on the pasture where the grazing horse eats them. After ingestion, the larvae hatch and develop in the wall of the large intestine before becoming egg-laying adults 4–5 months later. Eggs can remain viable for 12 months on pasture.

Bots (*Gasterophilus* Spp.)

The bee-like adult bot fly lays its yellow eggs on the hairs of the horse's legs, shoulders and neck during the summer months, i.e. July to September; when the horse licks itself it takes eggs into its mouth, the eggs hatch and the maggot-like larvae pass to the stomach, where the larvae mature before being passed out in the droppings 8–10 months later, i.e. the following spring. The larvae pupate and then hatch 3–5 weeks later as adult flies to complete the cycle. Traditionally horses have been treated for bots in the late autumn, after the first frosts, and again in the spring to remove any bots that did not pass out spontaneously. Large bot populations can cause ulceration of the horse's stomach. Ivermectin is the recommended treatment for bots.

Tapeworms (*Anoplocephala perfoliata*)

The adult tapeworm is found in the caecum and favours the ileocaecal junction, where the small intestine enters the caecum. The adult is segmented and about 8 cm long and 8–14 mm wide; it sheds segments containing eggs which are passed out in the dung. Eggs are eaten by an intermediate host, forage mites, where larval development takes place. The horse is infected by eating these mites while grazing and the larval form develops directly to the adult worm in the caecum, taking 6–10 weeks. Infection has been associated with colics, peritonitis and digestive upsets due to inflammation of the gut around the area of attachment. Few wormers are effective against tapeworms and it may be advisable to treat foals and adult horses (but not tested as suitable for treating stallions and pregnant mares) once or twice a year with an effective wormer such as pyrantel at double the routine dose. Horses that have year-round access to grass should be wormed at 6 monthly intervals (March and September), while horses that are stabled during the winter should be treated 10 weeks after the grazing season begins (about July) and again in October before being brought in for the winter. It may also be a wise precaution to dose new horses for tapeworm.

Treatment and control of worms

Correct and efficient use of anthelmintics or wormers is vital to good stable and grassland management. Table 7.2 shows the drugs available for the control of worms.

Table 7.2   Drugs available for the control of worms.

Trade name	Manufacturer	Active ingredient
Benzimidazole drugs for roundworms		
Panacur	Hoechst	Fenbendazole
Panacur Equine Guard	Hoechst	Fenbendazole
Telmin	Janssen Pharmaceutical	Mebendazole
Other compounds for roundworms		
Strongid-P	Pfizer	Pyrantel embonate
Pyratape P	Hoechst	Pyrantel embonate
Eqvalan	Merck Sharp & Dohme	Ivermectin
Furexel	Janssen Pharmaceutical	Ivermectin

- Depending on the wormer used horses should be wormed every 4–10 weeks in order to suppress worm egg output and to minimise the migrating larval stages in the tissues. This applies equally to the pony out all year round and to the eventer or racehorse that only has short spells out at grass. Ivermectin has greater persistence in the horse's gut and can be used every 8–10 weeks, while the other groups of drugs should be used every 4–6 weeks.
- There should be a change over to a chemically unrelated wormer every 12 months in an effort to prevent the worms building up a resistance to one product. Small redworms have been shown to

develop resistance to wormers containing the benzimidazole group of chemicals; this group includes fenbendazole, mebendazole, febantel, oxibendazole, oxfendazole and thiabendazole. Once worms have developed resistance to one of the benzimidazole group they commonly show resistance to other wormers from the same group, and once resistance is shown it is not lost even if the wormer is changed; this means that benzimidazole wormers should not be used for small redworms.

- It is important to have a dung sample analysed once a year. If you have wormed regularly as advised and yet the horse is still passing out large numbers of eggs it is likely that the worms have become resistant to the chemical in the product that you are using. Resistance is more likely to occur if all the horses in a yard have been wormed frequently with a benzimidazole wormer, particularly if the paddocks are 'horse sick'.

- Good grassland management will help control the free-living stage of the parasites; appropriate techniques include ploughing and reseeding, rest and rotation, removal of droppings, harrowing and topping. Paddocks should not be overstocked with horses and grazing with sheep and cattle will help reduce pasture contamination.

- All horses should be wormed prior to turnout and before introducing them to fresh pasture. The treated horses should be kept in for 24 hours after worming so that the worm eggs which are passed out go on the muck heap not on the paddock. It is recommended that all horses grazing the same field are wormed at the same time.

- Regular worming is most important when the weather is warm and damp as these are ideal conditions for large numbers of larvae to hatch from the eggs on the grass. A wormer active against bots should be incorporated into the programme at the appropriate time.

In order for a worming programme to be effective you have to choose the right wormer at the right time. Table 7.3 shows the types of worms that affect the horse throughout its life and which wormers are effective. The guidelines given in Table 7.3 are the manufacturers' recommendations for the most effective worming programme. However, different yards have different requirements; two horses turned out

Table 7.3   Which wormer to use.

Parasite	Drug/wormer	Comment
Threadworms		
Foals 1–4 weeks old	Ivermectin (Eqvalan) Fenbendazole (Panacur)	Requires high dose: 25 ml ('half-a-syringe')
Ascarids		
Foals 4 weeks to 6 months old	Ivermectin (Eqvalan) Pyrantel (Strongid-P) Fenbendazole (Panacur)	Dose every 4–6 weeks Dose every 8–10 weeks Requires high dose rate
Large and small redworms		
Adults	Fenbendazole (Panacur) Pyrantel (Strongid-P and Pyratape P) Ivermectin (Eqvalan or Furexel)	Every 4–6 weeks Every 8–10 weeks Does not kill the eggs
Encysted small redworm larvae		
All new horses	Fenbendazole (Panacur)	One dose a day for 5 days
Horse with year-round access to grass		Worm in February and November
Horse stabled during winter		Worm in November
Migrating redworm larvae		
All new horses	Fenbendazole (Panacur)	One dose a day for 5 days
All other horses	Ivermectin (Eqvalan)	Effective at normal level Three doses a year
Bots		
All horses	Ivermectin (Eqvalan or Furexel)	Worm in November or December
Tapeworms		
All new horses	Pyrantel embonate (Pyratape P or Strongid-P)	Requires double dose
Horse with year round access to grass		Worm in March and September
Horse stabled during winter		Worm in July and October

on 8 ha (20 acres) which they share with sheep and cattle will not need worming as frequently as horses turned out on sparse grazing which they share with many other horses. Table 7.4 shows a sample programme for horses with year-round access to grass and a suspected high worm burden. Table 7.5 shows a programme for horses with year-round access to grass but a low worm risk. Table 7.6 shows a

Table 7.4 Sample worming programme for horse with year-round access to grass and a suspected high worm burden, worming every 8 weeks.

1 February	Panacur Guard (1) (fenbendazole) to remove encysted small redworm and migrating redworm larvae
29 March	Double dose of pyrantel to remove tapeworm
24 May	Routine dose of either ivermectin, pyrantel or fenbendazole
19 July	Routine dose of either ivermectin, pyrantel or fenbendazole
13 September	Double dose of pyrantel to remove tapeworm
8 November	Panacur Guard (2) (fenbendazole) to remove encysted small redworm
22 December	Ivermectin to remove bots and migrating redworm larvae

Table 7.5 Sample worming programme for horses with year-round access to grass and a low worm risk, worming every 8 weeks.

1 February	Routine dose of either ivermectin, pyrantel or fenbendazole
29 March	Routine dose of either ivermectin, pyrantel or fenbendazole
24 May	Routine dose of either ivermectin, pyrantel or fenbendazole
19 July	Routine dose of either ivermectin, pyrantel or fenbendazole
13 September	Double dose of pyrantel to remove tapeworm
8 November	Fenbendazole (Panacur Guard (1)) to remove encysted small redworm and migrating redworm larvae
22 December	Ivermectin to remove bots and migrating redworm larvae

Table 7.6 Sample worming programme for horses stabled all winter, worming every 8 weeks.

22 March (prior to turnout)	Routine dose of either ivermectin, pyrantel or fenbendazole
17 May	Routine dose of either ivermectin, pyrantel or fenbendazole
12 July	Double dose of pyrantel to remove tapeworm
6 September	Double dose of pyrantel to remove tapeworm
1 November	Fenbendazole (Panacur Guard (1)) to remove encysted small redworm
27 December	Invermectin to remove bots and migrating redworm larvae

programme for horses that are stabled all winter and turned out on to grass in the summer. Note: when using ivermectin the worming interval can be extended to 8–10 weeks.

Part 2
Feeding the Individual Horse

Chapter 8
Practical Feeding

One of the most important principles when feeding horses is use your common sense. There are certain do's and don'ts. Sticking to the do's is good feeding management and will ensure that your horse stays in good health and gets the most out of what it is being fed.

Behaviour at feeding time

Like all animals, horses can become protective at feeding time; this is particularly true in the field where the horse may feel that it is competing with others and lash out or bite in an attempt to guard its feed. This means that the feeder must be very aware and safety conscious when feeding horses in the field and in the stable. All horses are individuals and will have different feeding habits; some are always greedy, knocking over feed buckets in their enthusiasm, while others are more cautious, eating only when the yard is quiet. It is important that the horse's handler is aware of these habits so that any change from normal behaviour can be reported and acted upon immediately; a change in the horse's eating and drinking habits is often the first sign of illness. Once a horse has settled into a feeding routine it is unwise to change the type, time and method of feeding suddenly. Remember the 'rules of good feeding' (Chapter 2).

Feeding horses at grass

Hayracks must be a safe design, such as that shown in Fig. 8.1, and moved regularly to prevent poaching. The design often used for cattle with a feeding trough underneath can allow seeds to drop in the horse's eyes and may have sharp corners on which a horse can hurt itself. Some of the round cattle feeders are useful (Fig. 8.2), but they must be of a

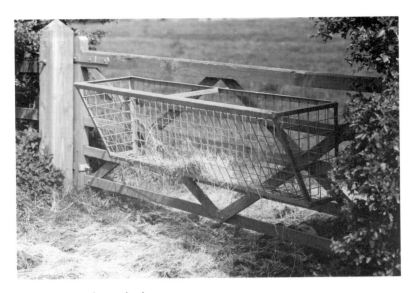

Fig. 8.1   Hayrack attached to a gate.

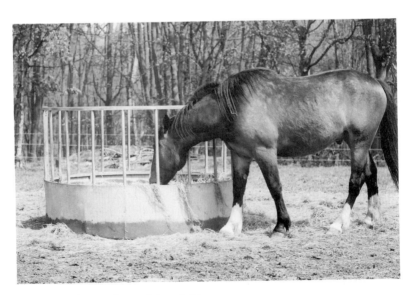

Fig. 8.2   Cattle-type hayrack in a field.

type that a horse cannot hit its head or become trapped. The rack must be heavy enough not to be easily pushed over when empty. Racks should be placed in a well-drained spot, away from the fence and with good clearance all round.

Haynets must be tied securely to a solid fence post or tree so that they will hang just over the top of the horse's leg when empty, or horses may get their feet tangled in them. Obviously this is tricky if you are feeding groups of horses as they will be different sizes; in this case hay is best fed on the floor – wastage is better than an accident. One more haynet or heap of hay should be put out than there are horses and they should be well spaced out so that kicking and bullying is minimised.

Concentrate feeding should be supervised as it is a time when horses can be very aggressive and accidents can happen. Always feed all the horses at the same time or take out the horse that is being fed and feed it out of sight of the others. There are a variety of buckets and troughs that can be hung over a post and rail fence although these can be knocked off and spilt. Non-spill feeders for feeding from the gound can be purchased, including those dropped into a close-fitting tyre. Some people feeding horses in yards tie up each horse before feeding it, thus ensuring safety and each horse getting its share. Feeding tubs should be spaced two to three horse's lengths apart to prevent squabbling. If one of the horses is new to the group it is best to feed it well away from the others. Feeders should be regularly cleaned to prevent sticky residue building up. It is useful if they have a drainage hole cut in the lowest point to allow rainwater to escape.

It is better to feed in a sheltered, shady and well-drained area away from the gate. This should prevent the horses poaching the gate area and mobbing you at feeding time. The feeding area should not be too close to the water trough and the hayrack, to encourage the horses to take some exercise. Some people prefer to change the area where the horses are fed to stop it getting too churned up. Others prefer to have one spoiled area rather than several scattered round the paddock.

Introducing a new horse

Horses have a clearly defined pecking order which has to be re-established every time a new horse is introduced to the group. The new arrival should be wormed and kept in for 24 hours so that the pasture is not contaminated with worm eggs. Then, if possible the new horse should be kept with one of the group overnight in a separate paddock to allow the newcomer to bond with an established horse. When the two horses are put out with the group the new horse will find it easier to settle and will have a companion to graze with.

Feeding the stabled horse

Most yards have a feed room containing secure, rodent-proof feed containers and a feed board stating how much and what type of feed each horse should receive in each feed. The quantity of feed may be expressed in 'scoops' in which case the amount of each different feed that a scoop holds should be known – horses should be fed by weight not volume. Some yards use a spring balance (Fig. 8.3) and the feed is weighed out for each horse. It is important that everybody understands the feed board and is able to make up feeds. All utensils used in the preparation of feed, as well as mangers and buckets, must be washed out daily. Hygiene is part of good stable management; it helps in the prevention of disease, and ensures that feeds will not be tainted which may deter a fussy feeder.

Horses may be fed in mangers built into the stable (Fig. 8.4), removable mangers placed in a bracket (Fig. 8.5) on the stable wall, plastic mangers over the door (Fig. 8.6) or in buckets on the floor (Fig. 8.7). If the horse is fed on the floor there is the risk of the horse pawing at the tub, tipping it over or fouling the feed with droppings. Any bucket used for feeding horses from the floor should be safe and strong. Plastic water buckets should have the metal handle removed; they also split easily if the horse knocks them about. Horses with respiratory disorders are better fed off the floor as this gives the airways a chance to drain. Some greedy horses spill their feed by pushing it over the edge of the manger or feed bowl. This can be controlled by anti-waste bars (see Fig. 8.5) across the corner of the manger or an anti-waste ring fitted into the bowl.

All feeders should have smooth edges to protect the horse from injury. If the manger is fitted into a wall bracket, the bracket should never be left empty as a horse may catch its leg in it. Sometimes the feeder may be a sink concreted into the corner of the stable. As some horses stamp or paw while they are eating it is a good idea to cover the concrete with rubber matting to prevent the horse banging its knees.

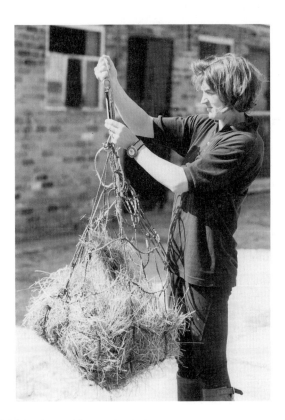

Fig. 8.3 Weighing hay with a spring balance.

Feeders should be placed where horses can see other horses while they are eating. Young and nervy horses tend to eat better if they feel they are in company. Many horses waste food by taking a mouthful then walking to the door trying to see others. However, it is important that a horse does not feel threatened when it is eating; this is often a problem in American-barn-type stabling where one horse can bully another through the bars separating stables. Nervous and young horses sometimes eat better at night if the stable is not pitch-black. A dim glow can be provided by a low wattage bulb left on during the hours of darkness.

Hay may be fed in haynets, hayracks or loose on the floor. Haynets allow a weighed amount to be fed easily. It is good practice to weigh the amount of feed a horse receives; there is less wastage and the hay

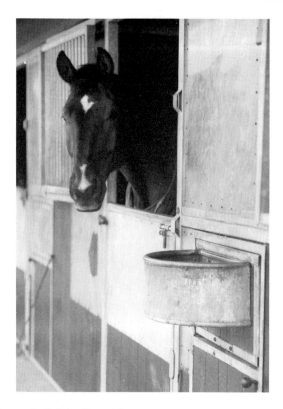

Fig. 8.4   Manger built into the stable.

used can be accounted for. A bale of hay weighs between 20 and 25 kg (44 and 55 lb) and usually falls into slices when the bale is opened; the slices will vary in size but often are about 2 kg (4.5 lb). Hayracks (Fig. 8.8) are easy to use but can be difficult to empty if the horse does not eat all the hay; this sometimes means that rejected hay builds up, becoming less and less palatable. Feeding from the floor is more natural and allows the horse to sort through the hay, but tends to be wasteful with horses treading hay into the bed.

Preparation of feeds

Bran mash

Warm bran mashes have traditionally been fed after hunting and on rest days as a laxative-type food. Modern thinking is that the laxative

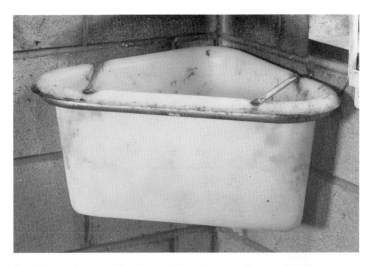

Fig. 8.5   Manger in a wall bracket, with anti-waster bars across the corners.

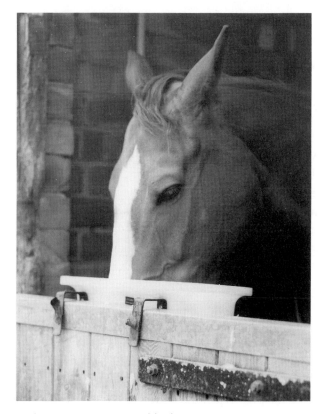

Fig. 8.6   Hook over manger on a stable door.

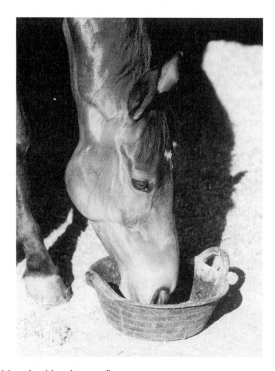

Fig. 8.7   Rubber feed bucket on floor.

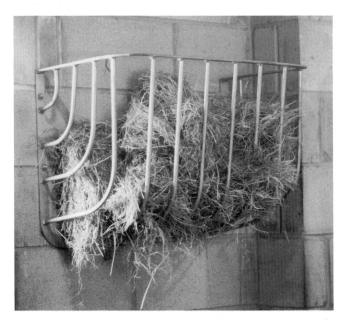

Fig. 8.8   Hay rack in a stable.

effect is minimal, only increasing the moisture content of the droppings by 2–3%. However, horses do seem to find a mash palatable and it may be a way to tempt a horse that is off its feed or to encourage it to eat medication. Bran has a poor calcium content and if bran mashes are fed, calcium must be added to the diet. Do not add the calcium supplement to the mash as it will not be utilised by the horse; instead add it to the horse's normal feed. To make a bran mash put about 450 g (1 lb) bran in a clean bucket plus a teaspoon of salt and a sprinkling of oats if the horse needs to be tempted to eat the mash. Poor on as much boiling water as the bran will absorb and stir well. Cover to retain the steam and leave to stand until cool. Correctly made the mash should have a crumbly texture. Molasses or cooked linseed can be added to make the mash more appetising.

Linseed jelly

Linseed jelly helps to lubricate the horse's bowel and improve coat condition. Linseed must be cooked before feeding it to horses to remove toxic substances. To cook linseed, cover it with water and soak for 24 hours, allowing about 500 g (1.1 lb) linseed per horse. After soaking, add more water, bring to the boil and simmer for 1–2 hours until the linseed is soft, taking care that the linseed does not stick and burn. Allow it to cool and add the resulting jelly to the horse's feed. To make a linseed mash, add 450 g (1 lb) bran to soak up the fluid after simmering and cover until cool.

Boiled barley

Boiled barley is traditionally regarded as an appetiser and an easily digested feed for tired, sick or old horses with poor teeth. It can also be used as a reward after competition or during cold weather. About 1.5 kg (3 lb) wet weight boiled barley can be added to every feed if the horse is lacking condition or added to a small feed for a tired horse. Soak the barley for 12 hours, then boil gently until the grains are just beginning to split and the water has been absorbed; this will take several hours.

Sugar beet shreds

Sugar beet shreds should be just covered in water and soaked for 12 hours. Cubes or pellets should be covered in 2–3 times as much water and soaked for 24 hours. Sugar beet should be freshly made up every day as it can ferment, especially in warm weather. Sugar beet pulp is a useful source of both fibre and energy for all horses; it helps the horse put on condition and up to 1.8 kg (4 lb) dry weight can be fed soaked per day.

The feeding value of grass

Horses grazing good pasture need little supplementary feed unless they are:

- Working hard
- In foal
- Have a foal at foot
- Growing.

However, adult resting horses may need extra feed:

- If the pasture is poor quality
- If the field is overstocked
- In winter
- In a dry summer
- In the spring when lush, spring grass may have a very high water content and a low nutritional value.

Feeding guidelines

Help your horse get the most out of its feed by following these simple guidelines:

(1) *When formulating a ration*, always start with the forage and add concentrate feed as necessary. Horses in light work only need a diet of good quality hay/grass with a minimum level of concentrates. As the workload increases the concentrates can be raised accordingly. Many horses are overfed relative to their needs. A minimum forage intake of 1% of bodyweight is needed to maintain healthy gut function. In practical terms this is 5 kg (11 lb) hay for a 500 kg (1100 lb) horse. If

poor quality hay is fed in large quantities the horse may develop a pot belly and lack muscle, especially over the top line. In this case the horse will benefit from a better quality ration combined with correct exercise.

(2) *Horses should be fed to maintain condition and performance.* However, horses differ in appetite and feed preferences and each individual horse's ration should be adjusted to suit its tastes. Remember, the feeding guidelines on a bag of feed are based on the 'average' horse and may have to be adjusted to suit your horse's requirements. Once you have found a ration that suits your horse, it should eat up with gusto; if it leaves food it is telling you that:

- The food is not good quality
- It is feeling stressed or tired, e.g. following travelling and competition
- It is feeling off-colour (not eating up may be the first sign of ill health)
- Its teeth may be sharp.

Horses may be tempted to eat by adding boiled barley, molasses or succulents to the feed. The appetite can also be stimulated in the short term by using vitamin B supplements or injections. If the horse is consistently leaving food yet looks well and has plenty of energy, reduce the bulk of the ration; you may simply be feeding it too much.

Some horses are allergic to certain feeds, coming out in bumps, having loose droppings or developing colic. It may be that minor allergies also affect the horse's behaviour and temperament. Rolled barley is often a culprit here; cooking by boiling, flaking or micronisation often seems to remove the toxic factors.

(3) *Try to stick to regular feeding times.* The horse, particularly when stabled for long periods of time, is a creature of habit and will learn to expect to be fed at the same times every day. Studies have found that feeding to a routine can increase the digestibility of grain by up to 40%. If the horse is kept waiting for its feed it will be hungry and bored and this may encourage it to develop stable vices. Work out a routine that suits your lifestyle and remember that punctual, regular feeding will help your horse get the most out of its feed. Some people deliberately feed their horses at varying times within a 2-hour period, so that the horse does not become too reliant on a rigid routine. If you

get stuck in a traffic jam on the way home from work you do not want to be worried about your horse going beserk, so perhaps it is better for the horse to be a little flexible. Punctuality of feeding is not as important if horses are turned out to grass during the day.

(4) *Feed the stabled horse at least twice a day.* The anatomy and physiology of the horse dictate that to keep the horse healthy it should have an almost continuous supply of food. Most stabled horses are fed hay and concentrates morning and evening, with some getting a lunch time and a late night feed. If you keep your horse at livery or work long hours it can be difficult to see your horse often enough. Plan accordingly, asking the yard or a friend to give the horse an extra feed. Feeds of hay and concentrates should be spaced out equally through the day, with the last feed containing the most bulk and the largest haynet to keep the horse occupied overnight. Ideally, a concentrate feed should not weigh more than 2–3 kg (4–6.5 lb) and should have a volume of about half a bucket; this avoids overfilling the horse's small stomach. Remember the 'rules of good feeding' (Chapter 2).

For example, a 16-hh (162-cm) horse receiving a ration of 5 kg (11 lb) concentrates and 7.5 kg (16.5 lb) hay could have the feeds divided as follows:

(1) *Turned out during the day*
    7 am   2 kg (4.4 lb) concentrates
                   2 kg (4.4 lb) hay

    Turn out
    5 pm   3 kg (6.6 lb) concentrates
                   5.5 kg (12 lb) hay

(2) *Turned out during the day*
    7 am   1 kg (2.2 lb) concentrates
                   2 kg (4.4 lb) hay

    Turn out
    5 pm   2 kg (4.4 lb) concentrates
                   5.5 kg (12 lb) hay
    9 pm   2 kg (4.4 lb) concentrates

(3) *No access to grass*
    7 am   2 kg (4.4 lb) concentrates
                   2 kg (4.4 lb) hay

Lunch time	1 kg (2.2 lb) concentrates
	2 kg (4.4 lb) hay
5 pm	2 kg (4.4 lb) concentrates
	3.5 kg (7.7 lb) hay

As the workload and the concentrate ration increase, a late night feed should be introduced.

(5) *Always feed the best quality you can afford.* Dusty and mouldy foods can cause respiratory problems and permanently damage the horse's lungs, especially in horses stabled over the winter. Handling dusty hay can cause illness in humans. Mouldy feed or hay can cause digestive upset and should always be avoided; do not be tempted to entice the horse to eat them by adding molasses. Dusty concentrate feeds should be dampened with water, soaked sugar beet pulp or molasses. Dusty hay must be dampened or soaked before feeding (see 'Soaking hay', this chapter). However, if a mouldy and dusty bale is opened it should not be fed, nor should it be soaked in an attempt to make it more palatable. Feeding poor quality hay means that the horse has to eat a lot of it to gain any nutrition from it, resulting in a pot belly and a poorly developed top line.

(6) *Always mix the feed thoroughly* to stop the horse picking out the bits it likes and to make sure there are no lumps of supplement. Dampening the feed reduces the dust and prevents the horse sifting out supplements or additives.

(7) *Once the feed is mixed and dampened it should be fed straight away*; if it is left it can turn sour and cause digestive upset. If you are travelling to a show, dry ingredients can be mixed and put into separate bags for each meal, but damp ingredients like sugar beet pulp should be mixed in just before feeding.

(8) *Leftover feed must always be removed and the feed bowl rinsed before the next feed is given.*

(9) *Feed by weight, not by volume.* Traditionally concentrates have been fed by the scoop, in other words by volume. If asked what we feed our horses most of us would reply in terms of scoops and have very little idea of the number of pounds this would weigh, let alone how many kilograms. The energy and other nutrients provided are dependent on the weight fed – your feed scoop should be marked to show the

volume occupied by 1 kg or 1 lb of the types of feed that you use. Use the kitchen scales and some insulating tape to calibrate your scoop. For the purposes of Table 8.1, I have assumed that a 'scoop' holds 2 l; your scoop may be different, but it serves to illustrate that if you substitute one scoop of barley for oats you will be overfeeding your horse by 5 MJ DE. This is not only going to have an effect on your horse, but also on your pocket; imagine that overfeeding being multiplied for every day of the year.

Table 8.1   Energy values of some common horse feeds.

Feed	Digestible energy (MJ DE/kg dry matter)	Digestible energy (MJ DE per 'scoop')
Oats	11–12	10
Barley	13	15
Maize	14	19
Extruded soyabean meal	13.3	17
Wheatbran	11	5

Forage should also be weighed; how many people know what a 2-kg (4.4-lb) haynet looks like? Horses are fed hay in 'slices' or 'wedges' which can vary dramatically from bale to bale. It is good practice and worth the extra time (until you get your eye in) to hang a small spring balance in the hay barn and weigh the horse's haynet so that you know the horse is getting what you calculated with the rules of rationing and not being overfed. A major cause of horses becoming fussy and not eating up is simply overfeeding. As a rule of thumb an average bale weighs 20–25 kg (44-55 lb). A 500-kg (1100-lb) horse on a maintenance ration and being fed average quality hay needs only 8–9 kg (18–20 lb) hay a day. This is only one-third of a bale of hay. It is no wonder that horses on box-rest and being fed to appetite to prevent them becoming bored often put on weight.

(10) *Feed to the fitness level required.* Plan your horse's feeding and fitness regime together; they go hand in glove. Overfeeding is just as bad as underfeeding and probably more dangerous to you and your horse.

(11) *Feed as few concentrates as possible.* Concentrates are not a natural feed for horses, and in excess contribute to problems such as

azoturia, lymphangitis and laminitis. The more fibre the horse receives, the healthier its gut will be and the happier the bacteria that break down the fibre. Very often as horses get fit they tend to ration themselves, and many racehorses and eventers are fed as much hay as they want and do not get a 'belly'. A problem may arise with the moderately fit horse, like the dressage horse, which is not doing fast work and does not ration itself and will get fat at the drop of a hat! The same is true of good-doers; these horses may need to have their hay rationed, but providing that you balance the ratio of forage to concentrates properly and then weigh both hay and concentrates, you should be able to keep the horse both happy and slim.

(12) *Monitor the horse's health.* Food alone is not enough to keep a horse healthy; exercise, routine teeth care and an effective worming programme are also vital. Your horse's droppings and urine should be observed and any changes noted. Use the amount, colour, smell, ease of passing and consistency of the droppings as a guide to the horse's digestive function, dehydration state and general health. Look for whole grains passing through unchewed and undigested. The volume, colour, thickness and smell of the urine is also a valuable guide to the horse's health and dehydration state. The diet will have an effect on the appearance of the horse's droppings and urine; Table 8.2 describes what is normal and possible dietary and other effects.

(13) *Make any changes to the ration gradually.* Sudden food changes can upset the horse's digestive system. Allow 7–10 days to change onto new hay or to introduce a new ingredient in the concentrate ration. Do not change or introduce new feeds within a few days of an important competition or event.

(14) *Always keep the food level ahead of the horse's workload.* In other words, if the horse is to have an easy day, you reduce the food beforehand. When horses come up from grass and start a fitness programme the concentrate ration should be gradually introduced, starting with small amounts, perhaps as little as 0.5 kg (1.1 lb) per day. As the workload increases gradually increase the concentrate ration by no more than 0.25 kg (0.5 lb) per day.

(15) *Reduce the concentrate feed on a day off.* To avoid metabolic problems such as azoturia the horse's concentrate ration should be reduced by at least half and preferably to one-third the normal amount,

Table 8.2 Dietary and other effects on droppings and urine.

	Normal	Dietary and other effects
Droppings		
Consistency	Contain 50–60% moisture; thus horse will pass about 50% more droppings than weight of feed eaten. Freely passed as well formed balls. No straining or discomfort	Loose, cow-pat-like droppings – green or wet pasture, excitement, worm burden, inadequate roughage Hard, dry droppings – dehydration due to excess sweating and too little water, introduction to dry hay in newly stabled horses
Colour	Depends on type of food and amount of green forage: Dark green – grass diet Mid-green – balanced hay and concentrate diet Light green/yellow – high concentrate diet	Very dark green and loose consistency – high clover content in pasture Very light green – high grain to hay ratio, eating straw bedding White, pasty – excessive grain intake, fermentation abnormality due to loss of gut microflora
Smell	Not offensive	Strong smell with dark colour – high alfalfa or clover diet Sour smell – excessive grain intake, fermentation abnormality due to loss of gut microflora
Texture	Well formed ball consisting of fine particles	Long pieces of hay or straw and whole grains – greedy horse bolting feed, sharp teeth, too much whole grain [over 4.5 kg (10 lb)]
Urine		
Colour	Yellowish and cloudy. Easily passed	Dark – high clover content in pasture, 'tying-up' or azoturia due to muscle pigments, dehydration due to concentrated urine, thicker consistency, small amounts

Contd

Table 8.2 *Contd*

	Normal	Dietary and other effects
Smell	Not excessive smell of ammonia	White/creamy – high protein, if also smelly could be bladder infection Abnormal – in grazing horses may be due to eating certain plants
		Strong ammonia smell – high protein in diet, dehydration Sour smell – bladder infection Abnormal – in grazing horses may be due to eating certain plants
Ease of staling	Freely passed several times a day. Some horses take more time to adopt the characteristic stance for staling	Reduced volume, slow to pass – dehydration Small, frequent amounts – urinary infection, mare in season Reluctance to stretch out – tired or sore muscles, dehydration

starting the evening before. The full ration should be resumed gradually over 2 days after work starts. The following shows a suggested feeding plan.

Work day before rest day

7 am	2 kg (4.4 lb) concentrates
	2 kg (4.4 lb) hay
Lunch	1 kg (2.2 lb) concentrates
	2 kg (4.4 lb) hay
5 pm	Normally 2 kg (4.4 lb) concentrates, cut to 1 kg (2.2 lb)
	Normally 3.5 kg (7.7 lb) hay, increase to 5 kg (11 lb)

Rest day

7 am	0.5 kg (1.1 lb) concentrates
	4 kg (8.8 lb) hay
Lunch	0.5 kg (1.1 lb) concentrates
	2 kg (4.4 lb) hay

5 pm	1 kg (4.4 lb) concentrates
	5 kg (11 lb) hay

Work day 1

7 am	1 kg (2.2 lb) concentrates
	3 kg (6.6 lb) hay
Lunch	0.5 kg (1.1 lb) concentrates
	2 kg (4.4 lb) hay
5 pm	1.5 kg (3.3 lb) concentrates
	4.5 kg (9.9 lb) hay

Following day resume full ration

If the horse is turned out for several hours on its day off and is receiving no more than 3 kg (6.6 lb) concentrates per day, it may not need to have its concentrate ration reduced.

(16) *Add fibre to the concentrate ration* to stop the horse bolting its feed and to help digestion. Fibre can be added in the form of soaked sugar beet pulp or chaff.

(17) *Although stabled horses appreciate having grass hand picked for them, lawn cuttings must not be fed.* Lawn cuttings tend to heat very quickly and can be bolted down with little chewing, leading to digestive upset. They can also contain foreign bodies and poisonous plants.

(18) *The horse should be given time to digest its feed before working*; it is recommended that horses are not worked for 1 hour after feeding. If the horse is going to do fast work it does not want to be full of hay or grass. Some people only feed half the hay ration in the morning if the horse is going to be worked hard and fast before lunch.

Soaking hay

Dusty hay can be dampened or soaked to reduce the risk to the horse's respiratory system. Sections of hay can be dampened by wrapping them in a wet sack for an hour or so. Very dusty hay should be fully immersed in a trough or tub. It seems that the duration of soaking is not as important as getting the hay completely wet. Thus, a 10-minute soak is sufficient provided that the hay is wetted right through. In many yards the evening's hay is put in to soak in the morning, and next morning's hay is put in to soak at evening stables. Clean water should be used each time as the dirty water will ferment rapidly in hot weather. Soaking hay in this way prevents the horse breathing in dust and harmful fungal spores, but if the horse is fed too much hay and it falls on the floor and dries out, the horse will again inhale the spores. If the horse has an allergy to the fungal spores or chronic obstructive pulmonary disease (COPD), great care must be taken in its stable management.

Chapter 9

Watering Horses

Water makes up 65–75% of an adult horse's bodyweight and 75–80% of a foal's. Water is vital for life; it acts as a fluid medium for digestion and for the movement of food through the gut. It is necessary for growth and milk production and is needed to make good the losses through the lungs, skin, faeces and urine. Restricted water intake will depress the horse's appetite and reduce feed intake, resulting in loss of condition.

Horses need an adequate supply of fresh, clean water at all times. The amount the horse will drink depends on:

- The moisture content of the feed, for example the horse at grass will drink less than a stabled horse on a dry diet
- The temperature and humidity
- Exercise
- Milk production.

Generally speaking a resting horse in a cool environment will drink 2 l per 50 kg bodyweight (0.5 gallons per 100 lb). This amounts to about 20 l (4 gallon) per day. Horses working hard and sweating heavily may need up to 70 l (16 gallon) per day.

Lack of water

Horses can survive for up to 6 days without water, but after 2 days they will go off their feed and develop signs of colic. A lack of water or insufficient water to make up for sweating results in dehydration, which upsets the horse's physical performance and metabolic function. Partially digested food in the large intestine acts as a reservoir of water and electrolytes; if this mass dries out impaction colic can result.

Water quality

Horses can be very fussy about their drinking water and water should be clean and of good quality. Most horses prefer to drink cool water and in the summer buckets should be placed in the shade and cleaned out regularly. In order to get horses to drink an electrolyte solution it is best not to add more than 1 tablespoon salt or mix to 15 l (3 gallon) water. An average size water bucket holds 15 l.

When to water

Generally, horses should have free access to water before, during and after feeding. Drinking will not interfere with the digestion or absorption of food. However, hot sweaty horses should not be allowed to drink freely. Once the horse has stopped blowing it should be offered small drinks at regular intervals until it has quenched its thirst. Once the horse is cool and dry it can again have free access to water. Some people offer water to the tired hunter on its return home with the chill taken off the water by adding warm water. During long distance rides horses should be encouraged to take drinks whenever they encounter water to prevent dehydration setting in. It is important that water should not be withheld from a thirsty horse at any time during an endurance ride. At the vet checks horses are allowed to drink as much as they want to aid recovery. However, under these circumstances, hot, thirsty horses are always given water that has had the chill taken off it. The hunter can be allowed to drink at a trough during the hack back to the box.

The horse at grass

Rivers and streams can be a good way of watering horses at grass provided that the river is running water with a gravel bottom and a good approach. Shallow water and a sandy bottom may result in small quantities of sand being ingested, collecting in the stomach and eventually causing sand colic. Ponds tend to be stagnant and are rarely suitable; they are usually best fenced off and alternative watering arrangements made.

Filled from a piped water supply, field troughs provide the best method of watering horses at grass (Fig. 9.1). Troughs should be from 1 to 2 m (3 to 6 ft) in length and about 0.5 m (18 in) deep. There must be an outlet at the bottom so that they can be emptied and scrubbed out regularly. The trough should be on well drained land, clear of trees so that the ground around the trough does not become poached and the trough does not fill up with leaves. During freezing weather troughs should be checked twice a day and the ice broken if necessary. They must be free from sharp edges or projections, such as a tap, which might injure a horse. If the trough is tap-filled, the tap should be at ground level and the pipe from the tap to the trough fitted close to the side and edge of the trough. The best method is to have a self-filling ball cock arrangement in an enclosed apartment at one end of the trough. Ideally the trough should be sited along a fence or recessed into it, rather than at right angles to it or in front of it. If not in the fence line the trough should be at least 3–4 horse's lengths into the field so that there is free access all round and horses cannot be trapped behind it.

The stabled horse

Stabled horses are usually offered water in buckets or automatic drinkers, both of which have advantages and disadvantages.

Buckets

Buckets can be placed on the floor, in the manger, hung in brackets (Fig. 9.2) or suspended from a hook or ring at breast height. They should be placed in a corner away from the manger, hayrack and door, but should still be visible from the door for checking. Providing water in buckets is time-consuming, heavy work and wasteful on water; they must be emptied, swilled out and refilled at least twice a day, and topped up three or four times. Horses frequently knock buckets over and may damage themselves by getting a leg caught between the bucket and the metal handle. They have three advantages: you can monitor how much the horse is drinking – a change in a horse's drinking habits may be the first sign of illness; they do not go wrong; and they are cheap – but the cheapest will not last long.

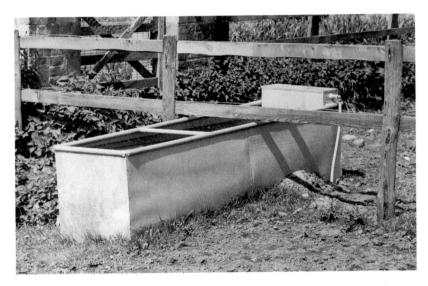

Fig. 9.1   Water trough positioned for access from two fields. It may be safer to place the trough lengthways to minimise the risk of injury.

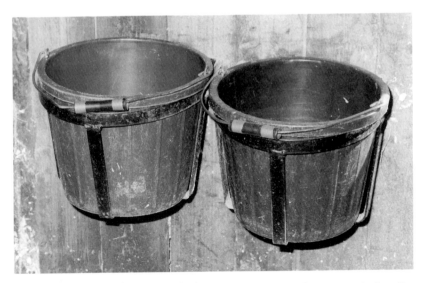

Fig. 9.2   Water buckets in brackets on a stable wall. It is safer to point the handles towards the wall.

Automatic drinkers

Although expensive to install, automatic drinkers such as in Figs. 9.3 and 9.4, are an asset in a large yard, saving time and effort. They should be deep enough so that the horse can take a full drink, and must be cleaned out regularly, sited away from the manger and hayrack and well-insulated to stop the pipes freezing in winter. Some horses are reluctant to drink from the small, noisy ones and water intake cannot be easily monitored. Each drinker should have its own tap so that if it malfunctions, or you need to monitor the horse's water intake using buckets, it can be switched off.

Water taste

Individual horses can taste the difference in water from different sources, often making them reluctant to drink when away from home. This can lead to dehydration and loss of appetite. If a horse refuses to drink, it may be encouraged by adding 2 tablespoons honey or molasses to a bucket of water. At home you can accustom your horse to drinking water with electrolytes dissolved in it after work or travelling. This will help to mask the taste of the water and rehydrate the horse rapidly. Highly chlorinated water may not be palatable to horses that are used to drinking river or rain water. If the water buckets are filled and allowed to stand overnight the chlorine smell will evaporate and the horse may accept it. If the worst comes to the worst you will have to take water from home to shows to encourage the horse to drink.

Some horses do not drink enough water, particularly when worked hard or fed dry feed. These horses can be encouraged to drink by adding electrolytes or salt to the feed. There are also horses that never drink at competitions; if you are just away for the day this may not be a problem, but if you are staying away the horse will become dehydrated. These horses can be tempted to drink by 'bobbing for apples'. Float a large apple in a bucket; as the horse tries to grasp the apple it will take in water. Eventually it may learn to drink the water to get to the apple.

The 'rules of watering'

- A constant supply of fresh, clean water should always be available.

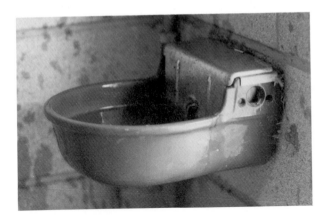

Fig. 9.3 Shallow automatic drinker.

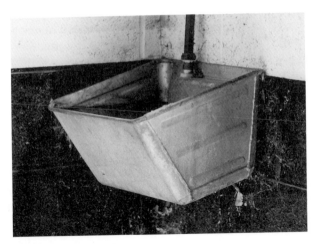

Fig. 9.4 Deep automatic drinker.

- If this is not possible, water at least three times a day in winter and six times a day in summer. In this situation always water before feeding.
- Water a hot or tired horse with water that has had the chill taken off it. (This is sometimes confusingly called chilled water.)
- If a bucket of water is left constantly with the horse, change it and swill out the bucket at least twice a day, and top it up as necessary throughout the day. Standing water becomes unpalatable.

- Horses that have been deprived of water should be given small quantities frequently until their thirst is quenched. They must not be allowed to gorge themselves on water.
- During continuous work water the horse as often as possible, at least every 2 hours. Hunters should be allowed to drink on the way home.
- If horses have a constant supply of fresh, clean water there should be no need to deprive the horse of water before racing or fast work. However, the horse's water can be removed from the stable 2 hours before the race, if thought necessary.

Chapter 10
Ponies and Fat Horses

Native pony breeds are usually very good-doers. They evolved to thrive in tough, mountain and moorland environments. This means that even on relatively poor pasture they are liable to put on too much weight. This is compounded by the fact that they may only be ridden at weekends and school holidays (Fig. 10.1). At the other end of the pony spectrum, some show ponies are more like small horses (Fig. 10.2) and need to be fed accordingly.

In most cases an adult pony in light work can maintain its body condition on grass alone during the summer. In the winter months, the pony will need to be fed hay and if the weather is very cold and wet a small amount of concentrates (horse and pony cubes) may be needed. Resting ponies can be maintained on a dietary intake of 1.5% of their bodyweight of good quality hay. Table 10.1 is a guide to feeding some

Table 10.1 A guide to feeding ponies. (The three ponies listed are examples that fit the bodyweight categories.)

Pony type and bodyweight	Resting	Light to medium work, e.g. Pony Club	Medium to hard work, e.g. hunting
Welsh Section A 250 kg (550 lb)	3.75 kg (8 lb) hay only	3–4 kg (7–9 lb) hay 0.25–1 kg (0.5–2 lb) cubes	3–4 kg (7–9 lb) hay 1–2 kg (2–4 lb) cubes
13.2 hh (134 cm) Riding pony 350 kg (770 lb)	5 kg (11 lb) hay only	4–5 kg (8–11 lb) hay 0.5–1 kg (1–2 lb) cubes	4–5 kg (8–11 lb) hay 1–2.5 kg (2–5 lb) cubes
Connemara 400 kg (880 lb)	6 kg (13 lb) hay only	5–6 kg (11–13 lb) hay 1–2 kg (2–4 lb) cubes	5–6 kg (11–13 lb) hay 2–3.5 kg (4–7 lb) cubes

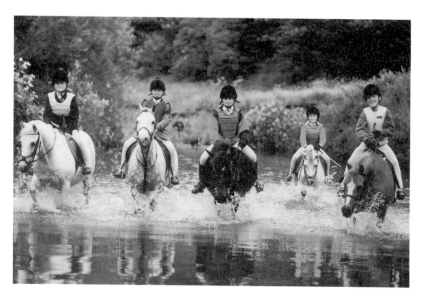

Fig. 10.1   Ponies at Pony Club camp.

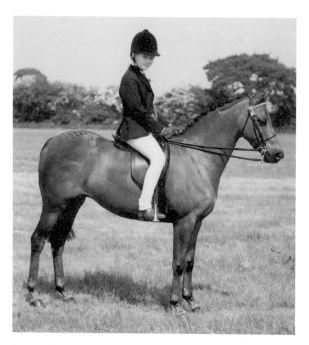

Fig. 10.2   A more 'horse-like' show pony.

particular ponies. A suitable concentrate feed would be a high fibre, low energy and low protein cube or mix. Many ponies can react to grain, becoming difficult to handle; this type of low cereal ration is unlikely to cause temperament problems or obesity.

In the spring, the grass contains high levels of soluble sugar and overweight ponies will be susceptible to laminitis. Feeding the laminitic horse or pony is discussed in Chapter 13. In ponies, laminitis is usually caused by a carbohydrate overload, for example eating too much spring grass or gaining access to the feed bin. However, there are other causes of laminitis, such as a mare retaining the afterbirth after foaling, and some ponies are simply prone to laminitis (Fig. 10.3). However, there is no reason why the recovered laminitic should not be fed and worked as any other pony (Fig. 10.4).

Slimming the fat horse or pony

Many ponies, cobs and Warmblood horses are overweight (Fig. 10.5). The amount of condition a horse or pony should carry depends on:

- Type
- Conformation
- Breed
- Workload.

For example, the show horse needs to be fatter than the hunter or event horse. Some animals become so fat that it becomes a health risk, perhaps predisposing them to laminitis and certainly putting greater strain on the tendons, ligaments, heart and lungs.

Obesity is said to reduce fertility of mares and without doubt can make foaling more difficult. Horses that tend to be fat are usually:

- Good-doers
- Greedy
- Receiving too much food for the work they are doing.

The problem is most common when the horse is only ridden at the weekend and, in order to keep the horse happy during the week, it is given as much hay as it wants as well as a concentrate feed.

Just as in humans, there is no easy way to slim down a horse. It must

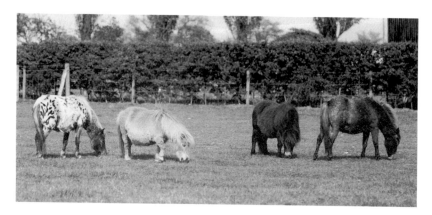

Fig. 10.3   This type of pony is prone to laminitis if not correctly managed.

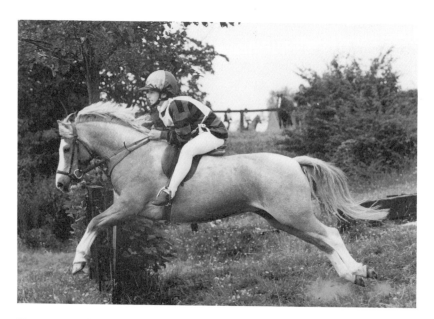

Fig. 10.4   With good management the recovered laminitic can lead an active life.

go on a diet and have more, controlled exercise if it is to lose weight. Horses and ponies should never be starved in an attempt to reduce their weight. Not only is this inhumane, it can cause serious health problems. For example, ponies suffering from laminitis which are suddenly put on starvation rations can develop hyperlipaemia. Pony

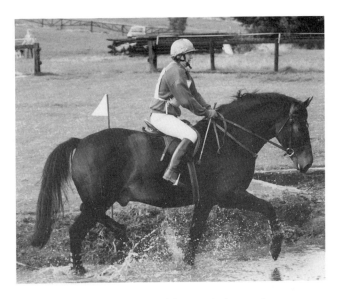

Fig. 10.5   Work is an important part of the weight loss regime.

mares in late pregnancy or early lactation that experience a sudden change in pasture are prone to this problem.

Workload

For the best long-term results the horse's weight loss should be gradual, accomplished by a combination of a lower energy diet and increased work. The duration and speed of the work can be gradually built up to include trotting, cantering and hill work. If possible the horse should be exercised twice a day to reduce the boredom factor. It is also an idea to give the horse a toy to play with in the stable.

The ration

The protein, fibre, mineral and vitamin levels of the diet should be kept at maintenance levels while the energy is gradually reduced so that the horse burns up body fat to provide the energy needed. The first thing to do is to cut the concetrate feed down to a minimum. If the horse is kept in a yard it will need to be fed at the same time as the other horses or it will start to bang its door and develop bad habits. For a 16-hh (162-

cm) horse with an ideal weight of 500 kg (1100 lb) the following ration is suggested to be fed three times a day:

1 kg (2.2 lb) dampened low sugar chaff
Either 250 g (0.5 lb) soyabean meal or one-third of the daily recommended amount of a feed balancer
One heaped teaspoon salt
Mineral and vitamin supplement [this need not be fed if a feed balancer (a specially formulated compound feed) is used].

The next thing to do is to reduce the hay ration. The horse should be kept on non-edible bedding and the hay fed in a net with small holes so that it takes longer to eat. Over a period of about 10 days the hay can be reduced to about 3 kg (6.6 lb) hay to be given overnight (the horse may be out during the day or being worked). This ration provides all the protein, vitamins and minerals that the horse needs but under-supplies energy. The ration does not satisfy the horse's appetite and a close eye must be kept out for the horse developing stable vices or becoming unruly. This is why exercise is such an important part of the regime.

Feeding straw

Feeding good quality oat or barley straw can be a useful way of providing the fat horse with fibre and bulk without oversupplying energy. Straw is eaten slowly and needs a great deal of chewing, keeping the horse occupied and helping to prevent the dieting horse becoming too bored. If the horse is at grass the grazing will have to be restricted, perhaps to only an hour morning and evening. The horse will have to spend the rest of the time stabled or confined to a bare 'starvation' paddock. The horse should get a small feed, such as outlined above, containing a mineral and vitamin supplement to ensure that the horse remains healthy during weight loss. It is possible to buy muzzles which allow the horse to only bite a tiny amount of grass at a time. This keeps the animal occupied and working hard for each mouthful of grass. It is a useful way of preventing ponies becoming too fat in the spring.

Chapter 11

The Working Horse

Feeding for maintenance

In the wild, the horse would spend the summer months grazing nutritious and plentiful grass, building up body reserves for the coming winter. A horse can eat 10% of its bodyweight in fresh grass every day. This means that a 16-hh (162-cm) horse weighing about 500 kg (1100 lb) would eat a massive 50 kg (110 lb). The reason the horse eats so much is that fresh grass contains much water so that every kilogram of grass only supplies about 250 g nutrition, so that eating 50 kg grass only supplies 12.5 kg dry matter. This is one of the reasons why a horse kept at grass drinks less water – it is taking in plenty of moisture as it eats.

The nutritive values of fresh grass in Table 11.1 show that it will oversupply the nutrients that the horse needs to maintain itself. Surplus energy and protein are stored as fat which can be burned up in the winter when the grass is in short supply. Grass is also a good supplier of ß-carotene which is converted to vitamin A in the body and stored in the liver. Exposure to sunshine helps the horse build up body reserves of vitamin D, so you can see that summer grazing and sunshine are invaluable for horses, especially if they are to winter out. Some working horses are lucky enough to be kept like this, but very often

Table 11.1 Nutritive values of fresh and preserved grass.

Feed	Dry matter (%)	Composition of the dry matter		
		DE (MJ)	Fibre (%)	Protein (%)
Young grass	20	14	20	17
Mature grass	25	10	30	8–9
Grass hay	86	7–8	30	4–8
Big bale silage	55–65	10–12	30	8–12

horse owners have limited access to grazing and the grazing is often overstocked and of poor quality. These horses will need additional hay and possibly hard feed, even during the summer.

Feeding for light work

Most people assume that as soon as a horse starts to work then it needs to be fed concentrates. This is not the case and many horses can do quite a lot of work without needing any hard feed. Another problem is that people often overestimate the amount of work that their horse is doing; just because you are working hard on top does not mean that the horse is working equally hard. Many owners have to try to fit their riding in around a job and a family; their horses may work fairly hard at the weekend but do little in the week. We want our horses to look their best and to be contented. As a result, many horses are overfed for the amount of work they are doing. This excess energy not only makes the horse fat but also can lead to temperamental behaviour and a lack of control.

The two main points that determine whether or not a horse needs extra food are:

- The quality of the hay. Poor quality hay may not even support a resting horse while good quality hay may enable the horse to work with very little extra feed
- The horse's bodyweight. If the horse is losing condition it needs more feed; if it is maintaining its bodyweight it does not need extra feed.

Obviously the horse will need to be given something to eat when all the other horses in the yard are being fed. This may only consist of a double handful of chaff and some carrots. Do not worry: you may feel guilty only giving a tiny feed, but to the horse a feed is a feed – size is not important.

Depending on the amount of grazing, a 16-hh (162-cm), 500-kg (1100-lb) horse will need about 7.5–12.5 kg (16.5–28 lb) hay per day. Depending on the quality of the hay, this will supply all the horse's energy requirements, but the horse is likely to be short of protein and minerals and vitamins. The adult resting horse needs about 10% protein in the ration; Table 11.1 shows that hay rarely has a protein level this high. This can be put right by feeding a small amount of a specially formulated compound feed called a balancer which is high in protein and fully supplemented with minerals and vitamins. Balancers can sometimes have a dramatic effect on the horse's condition when used to balance the ration as they help the horse use its feed effectively. Alternatively, a high protein feed, such as soya, dried grass or alfalfa, could be fed.

Feeding for performance

Successful performance depends on a combination of good stable management, feeding and exercise. While good feeding will not make a horse jump higher or run faster, poor feeding will undoubtedly damage a horse's ability to perform. Overfeeding or underfeeding will impair a horse's performance. A good trainer is one who can balance the horse's work and feed to produce an athlete ready to give its best. Generalisations are always a mistake; however, there are a few general guidelines which are the same for all horses, regardless of the competitive goal:

- Once a horse is receiving its full ration of concentrates it should be given at least three feeds a day. If the horse is not eating up, give a late night feed, so that it is receiving the same weight of feed but in four smaller feeds.
- If the horse is not put out to grass it should have its hay ration divided into three, with the largest amount being given at night. It is not good for the horse to go for long periods of time without food in its gut; if it is given hay at 5 PM and not fed until 8 AM the following morning, it may well go over 12 hours with no food, so try to make the evening hay ration as large as possible.
- The horse should have a salt lick in the manger. This will help to stop the horse bolting its feed and provide it with a minimum amount of salt. Many horses in hard work which are sweating heavily will not receive enough salt from this lick alone. As soon as your horse starts to do any hard work which makes it sweat, it should be given electrolytes in the evening feed or in the water.
- Fresh, clean water should be available at all times; drinkers and buckets must be regularly scrubbed out.

- The concentrate feed intake must always be severely restricted if the horse has to be laid off work. If your horse goes out in the field on its day off, the concentrate ration should be halved and the hay increased. If the horse has to stand in the stable without exercise for any reason, the concentrate feed should be reduced even more.

Energy

The exercising horse will need more energy; hard, fast work such as racing or advanced three-day eventing may double the horse's daily energy requirement. The energy expended, for example, by a hunter during a hard day cannot be matched by its energy intake of that day. Energy stores are replenished over the next 2–3 days.

Protein

If the energy intake is adequate then it is likely that the working horse is receiving adequate amounts of protein. The actual requirement does increase slightly due to the protein lost in sweat and the protein taken up by muscle tissue. While there is some argument about the relationship between protein levels in the diet and performance it is sensible not to overfeed protein.

Minerals

The need for magnesium, iron, selenium and iodine would be expected to increase with exercise. Magnesium is involved in energy release, iron is essential for the formation of haemoglobin in the red blood cells, selenium is important for muscle function, and iodine is necessary for general metabolism.

Vitamins

Vitamin E is considered important for the exercising horse and stress increases the horse's demand for B complex vitamins. Most compound feeds designed for performance horses will contain suitable levels of vitamins and minerals. If a cereal-based ration is being fed a supplement designed for working horses should be included.

Electrolytes

Electrolytes are substances that dissolve in the water within the cells of the body. Their role is to maintain the fluid balance within the cell so that the cell can function properly. When the horse sweats, water and electrolytes are lost. If these are not replaced the horse becomes dehydrated and the balance of fluid in the body is disturbed. The most important electrolytes are sodium, potassium, calcium, magnesium, chloride and bicarbonate. An electrolyte mixture should be fed or given in the water after the horse has sweated, not just after competitions. Thus, the hunter needs electrolytes after a day's hunting, the dressage horse needs them after a strenuous lesson, the eventer needs them after fast work and the show jumper needs them if it has sweated up on the way to a show.

Feeding show horses and dressage horses

Show horses and dressage horses (Figs 11.1, 11.2) are trained to have impeccable manners and to move freely and well. They need to be in very good condition with a gleaming coat, radiating good health. In recent years, Warmblood breeds have become increasingly popular as dressage horses due to their natural movement and trainability. While speed is not important, these horses have to be fit enough to cope with the demands of their sport. The show horse has to have enough stamina to still have plenty of presence at the end of a long day while the dressage horse has to perform strictly controlled athletic exercises. This means that while they may not do fast work, they have to be able to cope with daily schooling sessions without losing any condition. The feeding regime must also ensure that the horse is calm, well mannered and responsive in the ring. These horses may travel extensively to compete; this is tiring and they must not go off their food or dehydrate as this will affect their vitality.

The horse will need enough energy in the diet to keep it in good condition, but without making it overfresh. The amount and type of food will depend on:

- Temperament
- Workload
- The horse's individual preferences.

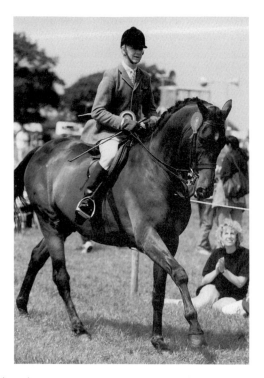

Fig. 11.1   A show horse.

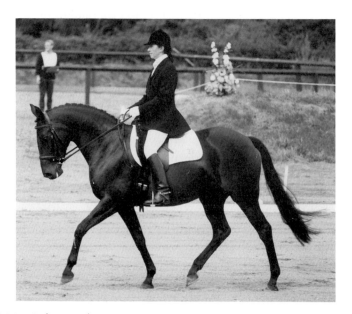

Fig. 11.2   A dressage horse.

Some horses become 'hot' when fed soluble carbohydrate feeds such as oats or barley and alternative ways of providing energy have to be found. Sunflower oil or corn oil is a useful source of slow release energy which can replace some grain and has the added advantage of enhancing coat and skin condition. About 275 ml (0.5 pt) oil has the same energy value as 700 g (1.5 lb) oats.

Some people use vitamins such as E and B_1 to maintain a stable temperament at a show, while others use herbal preparations.

The ration should be based on good quality hay or haylage and topped up with highly nutritious, high fibre, concentrate feeds such as alfalfa chaff, sugar beet pulp and cooked cereals. Cooking increases the digestibility of the grain and makes it less 'heating'. Traditionally boiled barley was fed for condition; these days grains are steam flaked, micronised or extruded. Putting condition on horses is discussed in more detail in Chapter 12. Getting a horse in show condition may take months. Racehorses that are purchased off the track are used to eating a low bulk, high concentrate diet. It may take them 6 months to relax or 'let down' and fill out into the proportions required by the show ring, to eat a larger volume of food and get the most out of a high bulk diet. As time passes, these horses usually relax and gain condition.

Dressage and show horses do not have a high requirement for protein and if the horse is receiving enough energy it is probably getting enough protein. However, if the horse needs building up it may be necessary to add soyabean, milk pellets or a high protein balancer pellet. As these horses are likely to spend the majority of their time stabled it is important for them to have plenty of fibre in the ration. The bulk of the hay ration should be given at night to keep the horse occupied and stop it getting bored and developing stable vices.

If the horse is on a grain based ration it should receive a broad spectrum mineral and vitamin supplement. Depending on the formulation of the supplement, the horse may also need a source of calcium to maintain the calcium to phosphorus ratio in the diet. This can be done by feeding 50 g dicalcium phosphate per day. The horse should also have access to a salt lick, but this is not a complete electrolyte replacer for a heavily sweating horse. During hot weather when horses are sweating up during travelling or training or at a show an electrolyte supplement should be used at the recommended dose. It is important that these horses drink at shows and during long journeys.

Care must be taken to cut the concentrate feed on rest days; this will reduce the risk of 'tying-up' (azoturia) and help control overfresh behaviour. If the horse is standing in the stable without exercise, the concentrate should be cut the night before the rest day and then reintroduced over 2 days once work has resumed.

Both dressage horses and show horses may compete very frequently with a long competition season. The skill in feeding these horses is to keep their condition and to keep them mentally fresh without over- or underfeeding them; it is equally important to achieve the correct overall energy content of the diet in these horses, as it is in racehorses.

Ration for a 16.2-hh (164-cm) dressage or show horse

- Limited period at grass every day
- Work 60 minutes every day, schooling and hacking
- Two feeds per day.

Oats	2.2 kg (5 lb)	Replace 0.7 kg (1.5 lb) with 250 ml (0.4 pt) oil if horse 'hots up' (becomes overexuberant).
or Barley	2.2 kg (5 lb)	Micronised or steam flaked.
plus Maize	0.9 kg (2 lb)	Micronised or steam flaked added if extra condition or energy needed.
or Competition Nuts/Mix	2.7–3.6 kg (6–8 lb)	Feed less of a competition feed or more of a 'cool' feed.
plus Oil	500 ml (0.8 pt)	Two teacups in each feed in addition for thin horses, replacing grain in hot horses.
plus		
Sugar beet pulp	0.45 kg (1 lb)	Dry weight soaked, to damp feed and add digestible fibre.
Alfalfa chaff	Up to 1.8 kg (4 lb)	To bulk out feed, a useful source of non-heating energy plus protein and calcium.
General purpose supplement		If on grain diet or 'cool' mix.
Electrolyte		To replace salts lost in sweat.
Vitamin B complex		Helps maintain appetite

Dicalcium phosphate		If on grain diet.
Hay	5.4–8.1 kg (12–18 lb)	Feed to appetite unless becoming too fat.

Feeding eventers, show jumpers and hunters

Competition horses undergo rigorous training programmes in preparation for competition. The stress of travelling, staying away from home and competing can wear the horse down as the season progresses, so while the energy demands of actual competition may not be that great, the wider picture must be taken into consideration. An added factor is that these horses generally have very limited access to grazing, being turned out for exercise and relaxation rather than to eat.

The event horse

The event horse has to be fit enough to gallop and jump at speed and yet disciplined enough to perform dressage and show jumping. This has led to many event riders trying to keep their horses happy mentally and physically by feeding as few concentrates as possible and turning their horses out in the field every day. The three-day-event horse may have a very rigorous training programme and yet only compete in a few events on the run-up to the main competition before being turned away on holiday, while the lower level horse may compete once a week throughout the long event season. These horses have widely differing feed requirements.

The one-day event horse

A novice event horse could munch on a haynet while being plaited on the morning of the competition; if the competition time is early, the horse should not receive any bulk while travelling until after its cross-country. If its cross-country time is late it could have a small haynet while travelling. Depending on your times, the horse may be able to have a concentrate feed between the dressage and the showjumping, providing that there is at least 2 hours' digestion time. The horse should be offered water frequently throughout the day and allowed to drink between the show jumping and the cross-country, even if they are very close together.

Ration for a 16.2-hh (164-cm) novice one-day eventer

- Limited period at grass every day
- Work 60 minutes every day, schooling and hacking
- Two feeds per day.

Oats	2.7 kg (6 lb)	Replace 0.7 kg (1.5 lb) with 250 ml (0.4 pt) oil if horse hots up.
or Barley	2.2 kg (5 lb)	Micronised or steam flaked.
or Competition Nuts/Mix	2.7 kg (6 lb)	Should be guaranteed free of prohibited substances.
plus Oil	500 ml (0.8 pt)	Two teacups in each feed.
plus		
Sugar beet pulp	0.45 kg (1 lb)	Dry weight soaked, to damp feed and add digestible fibre.
Alfalfa chaff	0.45 kg (1 lb)	To bulk out feed, a useful source of non-heating energy plus protein and calcium.
General purpose supplement		If on grain diet or 'cool' mix. Heavily stressed horses may need extra iron, selenium and vitamins A, E and B complex.
Electrolyte		To replace salts lost in sweat.
Dicalcium phosphate		If on grain diet.
Hay	5.4–8.1 kg (12–18 lb)	Feed to appetite unless greedy or inclined to put on weight.

The three-day-event horse (Fig. 11.3)

The amount of hard feed needed by horses competing at the three-day-event level can vary widely. The author has known horses go round Badminton on 3.6 kg (8 lb) hard feed, with plenty of energy to spare! These horses are supremely fit and if they are to maintain their composure in the electric atmosphere of the dressage arena, it is essential that they are not overfed. Some riders have to exercise their horses for

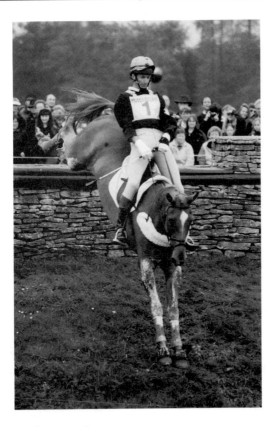

Fig. 11.3   A three-day-event horse.

prolonged periods prior to the dressage test to ensure sufficient discipline.

It may be that the fit horse needs less food than its semi-fit counterpart. It is harder work for the half-fit horse to perform the dressage movements and to gallop and jump than it is for the fit horse; the latter uses less energy and thus needs less fuel in the form of food. Look at the human equivalent: if you were unfit and did a 32-km (20-mile) walk, you would be very tired at the end of it. If you had trained for the walk it would be easy and you would not feel so tired. The author finds that fit horses usually limit their own food intake and do not overeat and become fat. Often a high energy food has to be given to supply enough nutrition when the horse will only accept small feeds. Again think of ourselves: the less you have to do the more you eat and the fatter you become. The busier you are the less time you have for food, the less you eat, the fitter you become and the less you think about food.

Many riders worry about the amount their horses eat during a two- or three-day event, but as long as the horse is eating its hay and drinking normally, there is no need to worry unduly. The horse has enough energy stored in its liver and muscles to see it through 3 days of competition. Prior to the event do not be tempted to change the horse's ration. However, it is permissible to reduce or omit the sugar beet pulp before the event or only reduce or omit the beet pulp on the morning of the cross-country day. If the horse frets away from home, reduce the quantity of concentrate food and use high energy, palatable ingredients such as milk pellets and flaked maize; generally though, it is better not to fiddle with the horse's feed too much as this may cause problems.

A three-day-event horse should have a concentrate feed no less than 4 hours before the start time of Phase A (Roads and Tracks). If it is competing in the afternoon it could also have a small haynet. Work being done on the timing of feeding and its effect on performance suggests that horses competing in the morning should not have a morning feed as this affects their blood sugar levels. However, until more definite conclusions are reached it may be wise to stick to the guidelines mentioned here. If the horse has had free access to fresh water there is no reason why it should have its water bucket taken away before it competes – why should the horse suddenly decide to have a huge drink?

The fluid and electrolyte balance is very important for the three-day-event horse and the horse must be watched for signs of dehydration. If a pinch of skin on the neck or shoulder lingers after it has been released and the horse has a gaunt, tucked-up appearance it may well be dehydrated; this really can limit the next day's performance severely. Ensure that the horse drinks and provide electrolytes in the food or water.

Colic can be a problem after severe exertion, and the intestines must be kept moving; once the horse is cool and its thirst has been quenched it may appreciate a small bran mash, with its normal feed later on. Tired horses are easily overfaced by a large feed, but dividing the normal feed in two and feeding it at intervals may overcome this. After the competition the horse's appetite will tell you how tired it is. Until the horse is eating up normally, it has not really recovered from its exertions and should be allowed plenty of rest. Hacks and grazing in hand (whilst led out in a headcollar) will help the horse relax and recover.

Ration for a 16.2-hh (164-cm) advanced three-day eventer

- Limited period at grass every day
- Work 60 minutes every day, schooling and hacking; fast work every four days
- Three feeds per day.

Oats	5 kg (11 lb)	Replace 0.7 kg (1.5 lb) with 250 ml (0.4 pt) oil if horse hots up.
or Barley	4.5 kg (10 lb)	Micronised or steam flaked.
or Competition Nuts/mix	4.5–5.4 kg (10–12 lb)	Ensure guaranteed free of prohibited substances.
plus Oil	500 ml (0.8 pt)	Two teacups in each feed.
plus Sugar beet pulp	0.45 kg (1 lb)	Dry weight soaked, to damp feed and add digestible fibre.
Alfalfa chaff	Up to 1.8 kg (4 lb)	To bulk out feed, a useful source of non-heating energy plus protein and calcium.
General purpose supplement		If on grain diet or 'cool' mix. Heavily stressed horses may need extra iron, selenium and vitamins A, E and B complex.
Electrolyte		To replace salts lost in sweat.
Dicalcium phosphate		If on grain diet.
Hay	5–6.8 kg (11–15 lb)	Feed to appetite unless greedy or inclined to put on weight.

The show jumper (Fig. 11.4)

The show jumper has to be well conditioned and responsive, without displaying excitable behaviour. Many jumpers are Warmbloods or have draught blood in them, making them more docile than

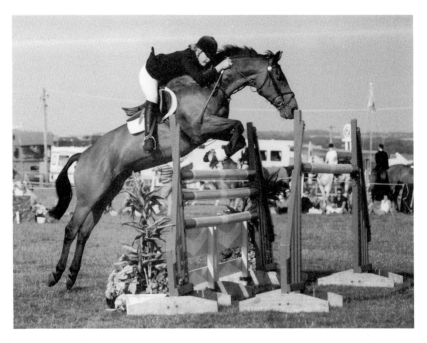

Fig. 11.4   A show jumper.

Thoroughbreds and event horses; as a result they are often fed more concentrates than their 'hot' counterparts.

Ration for a 16.2-hh (164-cm) Grade C show jumper

- Limited period at grass every day
- Work 60 minutes every day, schooling and hacking
- Two feeds per day.

Oats	3.6 kg (8 lb)	Replace 0.7 kg (1.5 lb) with 250 ml (0.4 pt) oil if horse hots up.
or Barley	3 kg (7 lb)	Micronised or steam flaked.
or Competition Nuts/Mix	3–3.6 kg (7–8 lb)	Ensure guaranteed free of prohibited substances.
plus Oil	500 ml (0.8 pt)	Two teacups in each feed.
plus Sugar beet pulp	0.45 kg (1 lb)	Dry weight soaked, to damp feed and add digestible fibre.

Alfalfa chaff	Up to 0.9 kg (2 lb)	To bulk out feed, a useful source of non-heating energy plus protein and calcium.
General purpose supplement		If on grain diet or 'cool' mix. Heavily stressed horses may need extra iron, selenium and vitamins A, E and B complex.
Electrolyte		To replace salts lost in sweat.
Dicalcium phosphate		If on grain diet.
Hay	6.3–7.7 kg (14–17 lb)	Feed to appetite unless greedy or inclined to put on weight.

The hunter

The hunter carries its rider for as long as 6 hours, spending periods standing still interspersed with short periods of galloping and jumping over varied terrain; it may cover 40–48 km (25–30 miles) in 1 day. This level of work may be repeated twice a week with the rest of the hunter's work consisting of gentle road work. Obviously the hunter cannot eat enough on a hunting morning to supply the energy it will use up during the day. This means that it has to burn up body reserves which are then replaced over the next 2 or 3 days. The hunting season lasts for about 5 months and it takes great skill to keep the hard-working hunter in peak condition. The task is made more difficult by the fact that the horse is unlikely to get out to grass, even for exercise, due to the time of year.

Traditional methods of feeding persist in many hunting yards, with a mixture of compound feed and cereals commonly being used. Horses are often given a hot bran mash on their return from hunting and before a day off.

Ration for a 16.2-hh (164-cm) hunter

- No access to grass
- Hacking 45 minutes every day, hunting twice a week
- Three feeds per day.

Oats	Up to 7.2 kg (16 lb)	Naked oats provide more energy.

or Barley	Up to 6.3 kg (14 lb)	Micronised or steam flaked.
or High Energy Nuts/Mix	Up to 7.2 kg (16 lb)	If a horse or pony or 'cool' feed is used (low energy), you will need to feed more to achieve correct energy levels.
plus Oil	500 ml (0.8 pt)	Two teacups in each feed.
plus Mixed flakes or flaked maize	1.8 kg (4 lb) 1.8 kg (4 lb)	Mixed maize, barley, peas and beans for condition.
plus		
Sugar beet pulp	0.9 kg (2 lb)	Dry weight soaked, to damp feed and add digestible fibre.
Alfalfa chaff	Up to 0.9 kg (2 lb)	To bulk out feed, a useful source of non-heating energy plus protein and calcium.
General purpose supplement		Heavily stressed horses with no access to grass will need vitamins and minerals.
Electrolyte		To replace salts lost in sweat – very important in the hunter.
Dicalcium phosphate		If on grain diet.
Hay	3.6–4.5 kg (8–10 lb)	Feed to appetite.

Feeding the riding school horse

The riding school horse needs to be completely level headed, healthy and to look well. It also needs to be fed as economically as possible without compromising its welfare. However, as always, quality must not be sacrificed for price. This nearly always is false economy – if you feed cheap, poor quality hay you may need to double the concentrate ration.

Good, clean, affordable forage is the basis for feeding riding school horses. In recent years it has become increasingly common for riding schools to use big bale haylage. This generally has a higher energy and protein content than hay (Table 11.2) and can dramatically reduce the need for concentrates. However, cobs and ponies may become too fat

Table 11.2 Nutritive values of bulk feed.

Feed	Dry matter (%)	Composition of the dry matter	
		DE (MJ)	Protein (%)
Grass hay	86	7–8	4–8
Big bale haylage	55–65	10–12	8–12
Barley straw	90	6	3.5

eating this type of forage and, rather than put them on strict diets which may affect their temperament, it may be better to let them fill up on some clean barley or oat straw.

Horse and pony cubes tend to be the concentrate food of choice; these are a low energy, low protein and high fibre compound feed. They also provide adequate minerals and vitamins for most horses and ponies doing 2–3 hours of slow work daily. Soaked sugar beet pulp is an affordable method of bulking out the hard feed. Molassed chaff, although easy to use, is an expensive way of adding bulk to the feed and provides little nutritional value. Older animals and more Thoroughbred types may need extra feed to maintain their condition, especially in winter. This can be done by using a higher energy and protein compound feed or adding barley, maize or mixed flakes to the ration. Remember that adding cereals to a compound feed unbalances it as it dilutes the vitamins and minerals; thus you may also have to add a supplement. There is also the risk that the quick release energy from the grain may result in frisky behaviour, which is not ideal in the riding school horse.

Feeding the endurance horse

Horses competing in long distance rides use up large amounts of energy both in training and during competition. As their job is to cover long distances at a consistent speed they need to be fed so that they have plenty of energy reserves without being fat. Indeed, this type of horse is often kept quite lean so that it does not have the added burden of extra weight to carry. It takes years to bring about peak fitness in the endurance horse, with most horses out at grass during the day and stabled at night. The type of feeding regime tends to vary depending on the breed of horse being used; many Arabs are very effective converters of food, needing little concentrate feed, while Thoroughbred crosses may need substantial rations to maintain condition and the competitive edge.

Slow release energy feeds that can be broken down during exercise to provide a continuous supply of energy to the working muscles are the ideal feeds. Thus, high digestible fibre and high fat diets are better than grain. During their training endurance horses have to learn to make effective use of body fat reserves as a source of energy and as a way of conserving the precious, limited glucose reserves. Once all the glucose stores have been used up the horse will become fatigued. Horses fed corn oil have been shown to digest it very efficiently and high levels of dietary fat slow down the drop in blood glucose during endurance work. It would seem that providing a high fat diet, containing 8–12% total fat, may stimulate the body to use it as an energy source, thus conserving glucose and allowing the horse to work longer before it becomes fatigued.

In practical terms, providing 8–12% fat in the diet means feeding 1–1.5 l (2–3 pt) oil a day. This is a very high level and although the author has successfully fed 0.5 l (1 pt) a day, more work needs to be done before this can be recommended. In energy terms 0.5 l (1 pt) oil is equivalent to feeding 18 MJ DE per day and means that you can reduce your concentrate ration by 1.5 kg (3.5 lb) oats per day. This is useful if you have a horse that is difficult to keep condition on or that tends to become very excitable on a high concentrate diet. Oil is digested in the small intestine, unlike cereals where starch passes to the large intestine to be fermented by the bacteria; thus, substituting oil for some of the cereal part of a ration may prevent the horse being as 'hot'. A high fat diet is also less bulky, which is useful for the smaller framed, Arab-type horse.

If fat is being used to replace concentrates in the diet, extra protein may have to be added, especially if the horse is given low protein hay and limited access to grass. The protein levels can be increased by feeding alfalfa chaff and a high performance compound feed. Studies suggest that additional protein may be useful after a ride to help the muscles recover. An extra 115 g (4 oz) soyabean meal can be added to the feed for 2 days after the ride.

The horse should be given plenty of fibre in the diet. Fibre traps water in the large intestine and acts as an essential reservoir of fluid which is used to replace sweat loss and to prevent dehydration during a ride. The provision of water to endurance horses is vitally important and they should be accustomed to drinking during the ride whenever possible; giving water little and often prevents dehydration without causing problems. Electrolytes are very important to endurance horses; they can be given in a horse's feed for a day or two prior to the ride and during the ride in water or sugar beet liquid. Sometimes they are given by syringing concentrated electrolyte solution into the horse's mouth during a ride before the horse drinks. The horse must be allowed to drink at least 4 l (up to 1 gallon) water after electrolytes are given in this way.

Ration for a 15.2-hh (154-cm) endurance horse

- Limited period at grass every day
- Ridden 16–19 km (10–12 miles) 5 days a week
- Two feeds per day.

Oats	3.6 kg (8 lb)	Replace 0.7 kg (1.5 lb) with 250 ml (0.4 pt) oil if horse hots up.
or Barley	3 kg (7 lb)	Micronised or steam flaked.
or High Energy Nuts/Mix	3.6 kg (8 lb)	Ensure guaranteed free of prohibited substances.
plus Oil	0.5–1 l (0.8–1.7 pt)	Two to four teacups in each feed.
plus Sugar beet pulp	0.45 kg (1 lb)	Dry weight soaked, to damp feed and add digestible fibre.
Alfalfa chaff	Up to 2.2 kg (5 lb)	To bulk out feed, a useful source of non-heating energy plus protein and calcium, helps soak up oil.
optional Soyabean meal	230–460 g (4–8 oz)	For extra protein if high fat levels.
General purpose supplement		If on grain diet or 'cool' mix. Heavily stressed horses may need extra iron, selenium and vitamins A, E and B complex.

Vitamin E and selenium		Important for muscle function and possibly resistance to 'tying-up' (azoturia).
Electrolyte		To replace salts lost in sweat.
Dicalcium phosphate		If on grain or high oil diet.
Hay	4.5–5.4 kg (10–12 lb)	Feed to appetite unless greedy or inclined to put on weight.

Feeding the polo pony

Polo ponies perform intense exercise for a short period of time and studies have shown that their energy and protein needs are similar to those of a racehorse in training. Many yards use a high energy compound feed topped up with varying amount of oats or barley to meet each individual pony's needs. Like all fit athletic horses, the polo pony should be in sleek but lean condition with a condition score of between 2 and 3 (see Table 5.2).

Ration for a 15-hh (152-cm) polo pony

- Limited period at grass every day
- Work 60 minutes every day, including trotting, cantering and galloping
- Three feeds per day.

Oats	5.4 kg (12 lb)	Replace 0.7 kg (1.5 lb) with 250 ml (0.4 pt) oil if horse hots up.
or Barley	5 kg (11 lb)	Micronised or steam flaked.
or High Energy Nuts/Mix	4.5–5.4 kg (10–12 lb)	Ensure guaranteed free of prohibited substances.
plus Oil	500 ml (0.8 pt)	Two teacups in each feed.
plus Sugar beet pulp	0.45 kg (1 lb)	Dry weight soaked, to damp feed and add digestible fibre.
Alfalfa chaff	Up to 0.9 kg (2 lb)	To bulk out feed, a useful source of non-heating energy plus protein and calcium.

General purpose supplement		If on grain diet or 'cool' mix. Heavily stressed horses may need extra iron, selenium and vitamins A, E and B complex.
Electrolyte		To replace salts lost in sweat.
Dicalcium phosphate		If on grain diet.
Hay	4.5–5.4 kg (10–12 lb)	Feed to appetite unless greedy or inclined to put on weight.

Feeding the heavy horse (Fig. 11.5)

There is a resurgence of interest in the heavy horse breeds. These horses are built for strength not speed, with naturally placid temperaments. They are generally good-doers, having a slower metabolic rate than lighter, Warmblooded breeds. Heavy horses require large amounts of

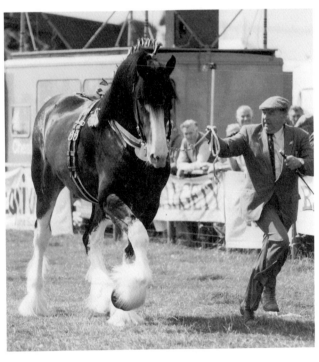

Fig. 11.5   A heavy horse.

bulky feeds and traditionally were fed large feeds containing a high proportion of chaff and bran. In most cases these horses will maintain their weight on good quality grass. If the grass is in short supply or of poor quality the horse should be fed plenty of hay. However, if the horse is working regularly or being shown it may be necessary to top up with some hard feed.

Although the traditional diet was oats for energy and hay for bulk, draught horses can be fed barley or compound feeds. A non-heating horse and pony cube is a useful basis for the diet along with a lightly molassed hay/straw chaff and sugar beet pulp. If the hay is of good quality a mineral and vitamin supplement and calcium should not be necessary. However, like all other horses, electrolytes should be given if the horse has sweated heavily.

Feeding the resting horse

Hard-working horses are often given a rest after the competition or hunting season. When this holiday occurs depends on the competition discipline. The length of the rest period depends on many factors:

- Age
- Mental attitude
- Any injury or health problems
- Time of year
- Competition discipline.

Summer

The hunter is lucky enough to rest during the summer and generally speaking goes out to grass looking lean and puts on condition at grass. However, if the summer is very dry or the paddocks are over-stocked, grazing may become sparse. If there is little shelter flies may pester the horse, reducing grazing time and encouraging the horse to walk off condition. The amount and quality of grass and the horse's condition should be assessed once a week and hay or concentrates fed if necessary. Vitamin and mineral supplementation should not be necessary unless the grazing or supplementary feed is of poor quality.

Winter

The event horse finishes the competition season in the autumn and is turned out just as the weather is turning cold and wet and the quality of the grass is falling. Even if there is plenty of grazing these horses are likely to need at least one concentrate feed a day if they are to hold their condition. It is also important that they have a well-fitting New Zealand rug. Frequently these Thoroughbred-type horses need more feed when they are resting in the field than when they are competing. A likely ration would be:

- 2 kg (4.5 lb) horse and pony cubes
- 500 g (0.5 lb) dry weight of sugar beet pulp, soaked
- 3 tablespoons oil
- 1 tablespoon salt
- A mineral and vitamin supplement at half the daily rate to complement the minerals and vitamins in the cubes.

The amount of grazing will determine how much hay the horse needs; generally it should be allowed to eat hay to appetite, which may be up to half a bale a day (10–12 kg; 22–26 lb).

If the competition horse has finished the season on the lean side then the concentrate ration should be such that it helps the horse put on condition. As the horse is able to exercise itself 24 hours a day it is unlikely that this extra energy will cause metabolic upset. If the horse is being fed a grain-based ration while at grass it should also receive:

- 660 g (1.5 lb) soyabean meal for protein
- Dicalcium phosphate (to provide calcium and phosphorus)
- A general mineral and vitamin supplement.

Letting horses down

Reducing work and fitness prior to a rest or holiday in the field is known as 'letting down'. If a fit horse, used to receiving a concentrate ration, is taken out of work, put in the field and not fed, it is likely to lose condition even if there is plenty of grass. Horses that are to be rested should be gradually let down or roughed off. Over a 2-week period the work and the concentrate feed should be reduced and the hay ration increased. The horse should be turned out for longer periods each day to accustom its gut to a grass diet. At the same time, the number of rugs should be reduced so that the horse can eventually be turned out day and night without suffering any ill effects.

It may take horses that have been in training over 6 months for their systems to cope with the change from a high concentrate diet to a roughage-based diet. Very often these horses lose condition and muscle, picking at their feed and appearing to be poor-doers. Remember, too, that these horses will have spent little time at grass and have little resistance to worms. Thus, when they are turned out with other horses on contaminated pasture they can pick up heavy worm burdens very rapidly. All new horses should be wormed on arrival and kept stabled for 48 hours so that worm eggs are not released onto the pasture. They should then be regularly wormed, depending on:

- Stocking rate
- Time of year
- Results of a worm egg count.

Initially the horse should be kept on a concentrate ration similar to the one it is used to. This can then be gradually reduced and the ingredients changed over the next 2–3 weeks. The horse will be fit and its work level should be sufficient to match the feed that it is getting and only reduced as the horse begins to feel the effects of the reduced level of concentrates and begins to 'let down'. If the horse is not suitable for ridden work it should be lunged.

Chapter 12
The Problem Horse

Specialised rations and careful individual feeding are needed for old horses or those suffering from sickness or recovering from injury to ensure that they receive a balanced diet which is adequate to meet their needs. Apart from these obvious cases, horses also need careful feeding in hot and cold weather, when travelling or in poor condition. The fussy feeder, the overexuberant horse and the obese horse can also be headaches for their owners. This chapter gives simple, practical guidelines for feeding the problem horse.

The older horse or pony (Fig. 12.1)

Just as in humans, the ageing process is a gradual one; while some horses will feel old at 12 years of age, others are fine up to 20 years or older and ponies live to even longer. So, just because your horse has reached its fifteenth or sixteenth birthday you do not have to change on to a specialised veteran diet. Let your eye and the horse's condition and performance tell you when, or indeed if, you need to alter the diet. Telltale signs include the following:

- Older horses and ponies often fall away in condition during the winter.
- They may lose condition in summer if the grazing is sparse, even if they are fed hay.
- They may lose their zest for life.

Many old horses have lost some of their teeth or have sharp teeth which reduce their ability to chew hay, grains and cubes. Poor teeth also increase the risk of colic and digestive problems. Pain and discomfort from arthritis may stop the horse moving around and grazing freely as well as possibly reducing the horse's appetite. Heavy worm

147

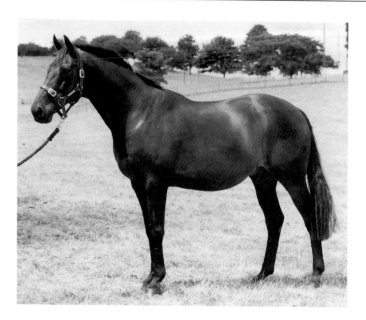

Fig. 12.1 The eventer Charisma in retirement.

burdens and overall reduced digestive efficiency in old horses may cause them to lose condition. As horses age their digestive efficiency decreases and they need more energy for everyday life; older horses also need higher levels of good quality protein, calcium and phosphorus in their ration. They seem to have less resistance to cold weather, worms, viruses and skin diseases. They need to be fed and cared for properly if they are to enjoy their retirement.

In order to maintain condition the feed needs to be:

- Palatable
- Easy to eat
- Nutrient-rich.

Feed manufacturers make mixes specially for veteran horses and ponies which are higher in energy and protein and with elevated levels of minerals and vitamins. These feeds are highly palatable, soft mixes, often containing alfalfa chaff, which are easy to eat. Alternatively, old horses can be fed boiled barley, soaked sugar beet pulp, alfa beet (a cubed combination of alfalfa and sugar beet pulp) or soaked alfalfa pellets. These feeds must be balanced by a broad-spectrum mineral and vitamin supplement along with 60 g dicalcium phosphate to supply calcium and phosphorus. Hay can be made easier to eat by damping it. If the old horse's teeth are so bad that it cannot eat hay, crushed, high fibre cubes or chopped hay should be provided as bulk. Old horses that cannot graze effectively can have fresh grass cut daily for them. During the cold weather old horses will need more concentrate feed; boiled barley can be added to the night feed or up to 300 ml (0.5 pt) sunflower or soya oil added to the ration. The horse should be kept warm by being stabled or rugged. If the horse is arthritic your vet may be able to prescribe pain killers to help it lead a happier life.

How much to feed

Table 12.1 gives some guidelines on how much to feed the older horse or pony. The amount of feed your horse or pony should receive will depend on:

- Size – smaller animals need less.
- Condition – older horses may be more prone to digestive upset; do not be tempted to overfeed. Putting on condition can be a slow process. Assess the horse's condition, grazing ability and the pasture value every week.
- Work done – older horses in work will need more than the resting horse.
- Time of year – as the weather becomes colder more feed is often needed to maintain condition. Stable or rug up the horse. In the summer, if grazing is sparse more feed may be needed.
- Condition of the teeth and feet.

Table 12.1   Guidelines for how much to feed the older horse or pony or one that needs to gain condition.

Height		Weight		Conditioning mix		Hay	
(hh)	(cm)	(kg)	(lb)	(kg)	(lb)	(kg)	(lb)
12.2	124	250	550	0.5–3	1.1–6.6	3–5	6.6–11
13.2	134	350	770	1–5	2.2–8.8	5–7	11–15.4
14.2	144	400	900	2–6	4.4–13.2	4–9	8.8–19.8
15.2	154	500	1100	2.5–7.5	5.5–16.5	5.5–11	12.1–24.2
16.2+	164+	600	1300	3–8.5+	6.6–18.7+	6.5–13	14.3–28.6

- Worm burden – ensure you have an effective worming pro-gramme.

Most manufacturers design their range of feeds to be compatible; veteran or conditioning feeds may make up all or just part of your horse's concentrate ration, depending on the horse's individual requirements. If you are in any doubt, ring the feed manufacturer and ask their nutritionist to help you sort out your horse's diet.

The horse that is losing condition

If a horse in good condition starts to lose condition, the first thing to do is to ask yourself why?

Health check

Before changing the diet you must check that your horse is healthy. If it is losing condition because it is not well, changing its diet is unlikely to help. Horses most often lose condition because of:

- Sharp teeth – the teeth should be checked every 6 months and any sharp edges rasped away.
- A worm burden – a regular, effective worming programme is essential.
- Pain – older horses may be arthritic; younger animals may have a back problem or sore muscles.
- Infection – horses can take a long time to recover from a viral infection; a blood test will identify this.

In addition to losing condition, the poor horse is likely to:

- Have a dull, rough or 'staring' (dull and lifeless) coat
- Perform below par
- Grow slowly (young horses).

These horses may not show an improvement in condition even when given extra feed. If they still fail to improve after 2 or 3 weeks, veter-inary advice should be sought.

Poor appetite

Alternatively, horses may lose condition because they do not eat enough to meet their needs. This may be due to:

- Mouth injuries
- Excessively bulky rations
- Unpalatable or poor quality food
- Sudden changes in feed
- Hard or fast work
- Fretting or loneliness
- Distracting or new surroundings
- Ill-health, pain or fever.

If the horse is off its feed because it is depressed by ill-health, pain or fever the vet should be consulted.

Teeth problems

Sharp teeth may cause the horse to refuse feed, become a fussy eater or eat slowly. Typically the horse rushes to its feed, appearing to be hungry and then eats very slowly, dropping partly chewed food out of its mouth (quidding). Young horses (2 to 5-year-olds) and old horses are more likely to develop teeth problems. The vet or horse dentist should examine the horse's teeth at least once a year and rasp if necessary.

Fussy feeders

Horses are notorious for having individual preferences for different types of feed. Do not make sudden changes in the horse's feed; this can cause digestive upset and put the fussy feeder off its feed. Indeed, one of the traps the concerned owner falls into is to offer the fussy feeder different feeds in an effort to tempt it to eat. This probably has the effect of putting the horse off even more. All feed changes, including supplements, should be made gradually over 7–10 days. If the horse is being put off by a supplement added to the feed, try mixing it with water and giving it over the tongue like a worming paste.

Unpalatable foods

The food may be genuinely unpalatable to the horse due to poor quality or poor storage. Mouldy hay or out-of-date feed should not fed or made to be more palatable by the addition of molasses.

Psychological factors

Worry will stop horses eating. Young or nervy horses can be distracted from eating by new surroundings, noisy stable routine or new arrivals in the yard. Colts or horses separated from their 'friends' may walk the fence line instead of eating and lose condition. Horses kept on their own and lacking the example of a companion may not eat as much. Some horses have a lamb, rabbit or chicken to keep them company.

Concentrating the ration

If the horse has a small appetite and does not eat all its feed it is a good idea to concentrate the ration so that each mouthful is highly nutritious. This can be done by adding oil and using a high performance feed, thus reducing the amount of feed but still providing equivalent energy and protein.

Poor appetite after work

Many horses suffer a temporary loss of appetite after hard work, particularly if they have become overexcited (e.g. hunting) or are unfit. It is likely that this is due to:

- Stress
- Tiredness
- Sore muscles.

It is important that horses are fit enough for the work they do and that they are warmed up and cooled down properly. Electrolytes should be used in horses that have sweated to replace the lost salts. Regular turnout also helps keep horses in hard work 'sweet', i.e. eating and happy in themselves. If this is not possible, grazing in hand or cutting grass for the horse will also help maintain its appetite. Some people advocate the use of B vitamin complex supplements to maintain the appetite of fit horses, especially those on grain-based rations.

The thin horse

If a horse arrives in your yard in very poor condition, do no be tempted to try to fatten it up as quickly as possible. The first thing to do is to assess the horse's health. The horse should be wormed, its teeth examined and it should be allowed to eat as much good quality hay as it wants. It may be wise to ask your vet to check the horse for any medical reason for its loss of condition and to take a blood test to determine if the horse is anaemic or suffering from bacterial or viral infection. Until these problems are sorted the horse will not thrive. Of course, the horse may be healthy and simply undernourished; this is often seen in aged horses and thoroughbreds that have thrown out of training and wintered on poor pasture. Other horses that may become thin include hyperactive types, horses with stable vices, and those that have been bullied and not allowed to eat.

Once the cause of the weight loss has been identified and treated the horse can be gradually given a higher energy ration so that it can start to put on condition. If possible the horse should be turned out to graze and for exercise every day. This will help the horse keep its appetite, avoid metabolic upset and maintain its temperament. Initially the horse may be too weak to be ridden in which case it can be led out in hand or quietly lunged for a few minutes every day. As the horse grows stronger, ridden walking work can begin; this will help build the correct muscles.

The concentrate feed should be increased vey gradually to avoid digestive upset and metabolic problems. A high digestible fibre diet seems to have the best long-term results while reducing the hyperactive behaviour often associated with the horse beginning to feel 'well' again. A ration based on sugar beet pulp and alfalfa chaff, with good quality horse and pony cubes added as necessary, along with *ad libitum* good quality hay, has proved successful. Probiotics, salt and broad-spectrum mineral, vitamin and trace element supplements will help ensure health. Some feed manufacturers have conditioning diets based on these principles.

What to look for in a conditioning diet

In order to grow fatter, the horse must be given more energy than it can use; the excess is then laid down as fat. The problem is how to over-supply the energy without the horse becoming overexuberant or 'hot'. The best way to supply 'non-heating' energy is by:

- Oil – look for a feed with over 4% oil
- Digestible fibre – slow release energy
- Cooked cereals for ease of digestion.

Also look for:

- Good quality protein to build muscle
- A full spectrum of minerals and vitamins.

Table 12.1 gives some guidelines for how much to feed a horse or pony that needs to gain condition. Above all, remember that all horses and ponies are individuals and must be fed as such. Any manufacturer's feeding recommendations are only a guide and must be adjusted to suit your horse.

Feeding horses in hot weather and dry conditions

Horses working and sweating in hot conditions can suffer from heat stress and dehydration which will affect performance.

The 'heating' effect of food

During the process of digestion and nutrient absorption some of the energy in the food is lost as heat. We are all aware of the effects of eating a large meal – a warm feeling of contentment and a strong desire to fall asleep! The fibre content of the feed determines how much of the energy is digested and how much is lost as heat. For example, the energy in cereals is up to 90% digestible, while the energy in roughage may only be 30% digestible, the rest being lost as heat. The heat produced during digestion can have a considerable effect on the amount of heat that the working horse has to get rid of, in addition to the heat produced by the working muscles. This heat production is a quite separate issue to the 'heating' effect of grain on the horse's temperament.

The ration can be modified to reduce the amount of heat the horse produces during the digestive process. Fermentation of fibre and roughage in the large intestine produces heat; while this is useful for the out-wintered horse, it increases the amount of heat that needs to be lost by the working horse. This can be a disadvantage for horses working in hot weather. However, the fibre in the large intestine acts as a reservoir, trapping water in the gut which is useful for heavily sweating horses. A balance has to reached, and the total amount of roughage should never be less than 50% of the ration. For the competition horse, the concentrate ration can be adjusted to consist of high energy, low fibre feeds such as oil, maize or high energy mix. This gives a smaller volume of low fibre feed with a high energy value which produces less heat. The majority of the roughage part of the ration should be fed in the cool of the day and when the humidity is lowest. Soaking the hay will help ensure that the horse is receiving an adequate fluid intake.

Feeding horses in cold weather

Bad weather increases the horse's energy requirements because it loses heat. It has been estimated that winter weather can double the horse's energy requirement. However, providing a field shelter and a good New Zealand rug (Fig. 12.2) can help reduce this need for extra energy. The heating effect of a high roughage diet can be used to good effect when feeding horses in cold weather. Adult, resting horses at grass should be provided with good quality hay during the autumn and winter when the grass is providing little or no nourishment. Depending on the amount of grazing, a 16-hh (162-cm) 500-kg (1100-lb) horse will need about 7.5–12.5 kg (16.5–28 lb) hay per day. Depending on the quality of the hay, this will supply all the horse's energy requirements, but the horse is likely to be short of protein and minerals and vitamins. This can be put right by feeding a small amount of a specially formulated compound feed called a balancer which is high in protein and fully supplemented with minerals and vitamins.

Horses thrive well in cold conditions; however, if the weather is wet and windy, or if the horse is losing condition, extra energy should be

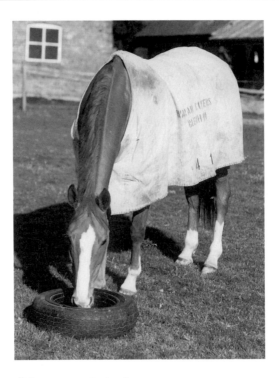

Fig. 12.2   A well-fitting New Zealand rug.

provided in the from of concentrates. A high fibre feed such as oats or high fibre cubes will provide extra energy to maintain warmth during cold, wet weather. If oats are used the horse should also be given a supplement. A resting horse might require about 2.5 kg (5.5 lb) feed in addition to hay. This should be given in two feeds a day whenever possible. Cold, hungry horses may bolt their feed so it is important to avoid giving them a large feed or, alternatively, to give them some hay first to take the edge off their appetite. Out-wintered horses should be fed in a sheltered spot as they will stand eating for some time and reducing the chill factor is important in maintaining condition. A well-fitting, waterproof rug will help keep the horse warm and dry, although a poorly fitting rug is probably more of a hindrance than a help.

Working horses will require extra energy for the amount of work they are doing; this can be supplied by cereals or compound feed, depending on individual preference. Horses in work and aged horses will benefit from either having an extra rug on at night or being stabled at night.

The fussy feeder

Each horse will have feeds that it prefers and it is useful to know which feeds and flavours your horse likes. This means that if your horse goes off its feed you will know what to tempt it with. Remember that horses rely on their sense of smell to accept food and slight changes in the smell, undetectable by us, may result in the horse rejecting the food. We have all added worming granules to the feed, or a new supplement, only to find that the horse refuses to touch it. Most supplements and wormers are flavoured to increase palatability, but the fact that there is a different smell may be enough to put the horse off. It would seem that most horses like aniseed, peppermint, vanilla, yucca and apple flavours and most will accept garlic in the feed. You can often train a horse to accept a flavour by smearing a couple of drops of the flavouring in the horse's nostrils or on the tip of its tongue for a couple of days. After this the horse will accept the flavour in its feed. Vanilla essence (5–10 drops) or garlic added to the feed may help tempt the fussy feeder. A tablespoon of salt may also improve palatability. Most horses seem to have a sweet tooth, relishing the addition of diluted molasses to the feed. Feed manufacturers add molasses or syrup to mixes and cubes to enhance the palatability of the feed. However, sweeteners must not be used to disguise the taste of poor quality feeds. Fussy feeders may be tempted by boiled barley, a bran and linseed mash or by turning them out to graze and relax for part of the day.

Horses can also be fussy about their hay; they tend to prefer good quality, leafy hay to stemmy, fibrous hay. Dampening or soaking hay can improve its palatability as well as reducing the dust content. Most will accept chopped hay or chaff, although some horses refuse alfalfa chaff.

The travelling horse

Travelling is a stressful experience for horses; during long journeys their feeding, exercise and sleeping routines are all interrupted. Fit horses on high levels of concentrates need special care. One of the major problems horses experience when travelling long distances is dehydration, so it is very important to offer the horse water at frequent intervals. If the horse is sweating it is wise to include some electrolytes in the water or feed. Some horses are more fussy about water than they are about food so take water from home in a couple of containers, so that the taste of unfamiliar water will not put the horse off drinking. If you have a real problem then try adding a little molasses to the water at home so that you can do the same at your destination and disguise the different taste. Fortunately most horses will drink when they are thirsty, no matter what the water tastes like.

The horse will spend a long time standing still during the journey and you do not want its legs to swell or for it to experience any other metabolic upsets; this means the concentrate ration must be cut down. On the other hand, you do not want the fit horse to lose condition. This dilemma is best solved by allowing the horse plenty of good quality, dampened or soaked hay during the journey, so that its gut is kept moving and partially full the whole time, so long as there are several hours allowed for digestion before asking the horse to work or compete; this will reduce the risk of colic and help hydrate the horse. The concentrate feeds should be small and easily digested and given at regular intervals. It may be useful to give the horse a bran mash the evening before the journey and only hay or a very small feed, including bran, the morning before setting off. If possible the horses should be unloaded every 4 hours, offered a drink and walked for 20 minutes before resuming the journey.

Horses should be allowed to fully recover from exercise before travelling. Thus, if they have taken part in a competition or race they should have cooled down, quenched their thirst and eaten before travelling home. This may even mean staying overnight. There have been cases of horses dying in transit after exhausting competition.

Horses with brittle feet

A significant number of horses suffer from poor quality hooves which are slow growing and crack easily (Fig. 12.3), leading to shoeing problems. There is rarely one cure for such problems; it is usually a combination of good farriery, correct stable management and a balanced diet, specifically supplemented as necessary.

Anatomy and physiology of the hoof

The hoof is a continuation of the skin, with the external hoof equivalent to the epidermis and the internal or sensitive foot equivalent

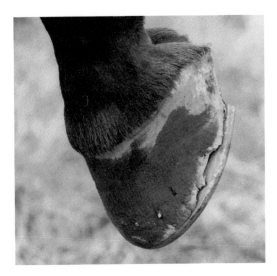

Fig. 12.3   A brittle, cracked hoof.

to the dermis or quick. The hoof receives nutrition via the blood supply to the coronary band and the sensitive laminae, not from the outside. Thus, hoof oils and creams can only have a limited effect on the quality of the hoof horn. It takes 9–12 months for the toe to grow from the coronary band to the ground, which means that it takes a long time to see any results of dietary supplements; you have to continue a treatment for up to 6 months to give it a chance to work.

There are many minerals and vitamins closely involved with hoof growth and, in most cases, it is unlikely that a horse is so deficient in one of these substances that it is causing poor hoof quality and growth. Important substances include the following:

- Sulphur is a mineral involved in the chemical bonds that maintain the integrity of the internal hoof. Organic sulphur which can be utilised by the horse (bio-available) is driven off by feed processing and may be in short supply in the diet. Supplementation with MSM (methyl sulphonyl methane) has brought about rapid improvement in hoof condition.
- Biotin is a B vitamin and studies have shown that supplementation with 15 mg biotin per day promotes hoof growth and improves the resilience of the hoof wall.
- Methionine and cysteine are sulphur-containing amino acids

which may be in short supply in the diet. They are the building blocks of keratin, the protein which makes up hoof and hair.
- Zinc is a mineral needed for hoof growth and skin condition.
- Calcium is needed for healthy bones and teeth and also has a role to play in hoof growth. Calcium is frequently deficient in horses fed a traditional hay and grain diet.

Despite supplementation, some horses still have foot problems. In some cases this is due to a fungal infection. This may be improved by topical applications which kill the fungus and strengthen the hooves.

For healthy feet your horse needs:

- Regular shoeing
- Good stable management
- A balanced, good quality ration
- Appropriate supplementation and treatment if necessary.

Horses with poor coat condition

The skin is the largest organ of the horse's body and the most visible. The condition of the skin and coat is a reflection of good feeding and the health of the horse. The coat should be glossy and shiny and the skin should be supple, gliding over the underlying structures. If a pinch of skin is picked up and then released it should immediately return to normal; any delay indicates that the horse is dehydrated or has a lack of subcutaneous fat.

As the skin is closely related to the hoof, any of the supplements designed to improve hoof condition are likely to help the horse's skin and coat. The bloom and condition of a dull coat will be improved by adding fat to the diet. This can be in the form of soya, corn or sunflower oil, cod liver oil or cooked whole linseed. A supplement containing vitamin A, iron, copper or zinc may be helpful and is said to enhance the colour of the coat as well as its condition.

The lazy horse

Some horses are lazy and in an attempt to encourage them up they are fed more. Usually these laid-back-types convert this extra food into fat, not energy, and as a result become even more lazy. This is a vicious circle which is very frustrating for the owner. In most cases the horse has to have more exercise and a less bulky, more concentrated ration. No one, including horses, feels athletic if they are full of food so the first step is to reduce the horse's hay ration unless its hay is already being rationed. The next step is to increase the energy density of the concentrate ration and reduce the amount being fed. For example, if the horse is receiving horse and pony cubes it could be changed onto a performance mix, reducing the amount fed by about one-third. Alternatively oats and maize can be substituted weight for weight for the cubes. Remember, adding straights to the ration dilutes the minerals and vitamins in the cubes and a broad-spectrum mineral and vitamin supplement and limestone or dicalcium phosphate should be fed. Some lazy, Warmblood-type horses respond well to a ration of racehorse cubes.

At the same time, the exercise programme should be stepped up, incorporating some fast work. It is useful to follow a programme designed for a novice event horse. Once the horse is feeling more energetic it will work more willingly; as it works harder it becomes fitter and as its fitness improves it is even more willing to work hard. Many late maturing horses will not reach this stage until they are 6 or 7 years old.

Chapter 13
The Sick Horse

Providing the horse with a balanced ration plays an important part in the horse's ability to fight illness, and correct nutrition is one of the body's defence mechanisms. Proper feeding of the sick horse should always be considered as an integral part of the nursing and therapeutic regime. The task of feeding the sick horse can be difficult and tiresome; the horse's appetite is likely to be depressed, swallowing may be difficult and the function of the gut may be disturbed. Any upset in gut function may lead to dehydration and a disturbance in the electrolyte balance, all of which are occurring just when the horse's metabolic requirements may be substantially greater. This means that there is often marked weight loss during illness, with a resultant decrease in the horse's defence capacity and prolonged illness and convalescence.

The diet

The sick horse's diet must have several special characteristics:

- Palatability
- Good quality protein
- Fibre
- Minerals and vitamins.

Feeding little and often is vital for the sick horse, with up to eight feeds a day, including first thing in the morning and last thing at night. Any rejected food should be cleared out immediately. Plenty of fresh, clean water must always be available, and it should be changed frequently. If the horse is using an automatic drinking system, close it off and give the water by bucket so that you can monitor the amount the horse drinks.

Palatability

Horses depend on their sense of smell when eating; if they have a respiratory infection, for example, and are unable to recognise feed by its smell, they may refuse to eat. Thus, the horse must be provided with the most palatable feed possible to encourage it to eat. Barn-dried hay is ideal if the horse has previously been fed poor quality hay. Maize can be gradually introduced into the diet; it is acceptable and has a high energy content. Molasses, vanilla, mashes and succulents can all be used, providing that the food is fresh. If swallowing is difficult the feeds should be soft and any carrots cut into very small pieces or grated. If chewing is a problem the horse may need a liquid diet.

Soaking or dampening hay may help and will also mean that the horse is taking in water. A smear of vapour rub in the false nostril (the flap of skin within the nostril) may mask the smell of medicines in the feed.

Good quality protein

The protein content of the sick horse's diet is more important than the amount of energy because the horse is not active and protein is needed for the repair of body tissue. Good quality grass nuts, alfalfa pellets, milk pellets, stud cubes, balancers and soyabean meal are all high in good quality protein; milk pellets have the added advantage of being highly palatable. Care must be taken not to overfeed the horse as it recovers or it will become overexuberant.

Fibre

Fibre is important in maintaining normal gut function, but as the fibre content of the diet increases so its digestibility falls and a compromise has to be reached. Molassed sugar beet pulp and bran are useful palatable sources of fibre and can be fed as mashes.

Minerals and vitamins

The sick horse may become severely dehydrated and it is important to supply a suitable source of electrolytes to help restore the fluid balance of the body. A supplement of minerals, vitamins or amino acids may be recommended by the vet, depending on the horse's blood profile. An anaemic horse would require copper, iron, folic acid and vitamin B_{12} as well as a normal broad-spectrum supplement. As always, limestone and salt are important.

Ailments associated with feeding

Choke

Choke is a term used to describe partial or complete blockage of the gullet or oesophagus. The blockage may be caused by the horse bolting its feed so that it is not properly chewed and moistened, the horse may be plain greedy or have a tooth problem making it painful for it to chew. Lumps of food such as apples and carrots can also become lodged in the oesophagus.

A horse with choke appears distressed and anxious; it may make repeated movements of the head and neck, arching the neck and then drawing the chin back to the chest or extending the head down to the ground. The horse usually drools and a mixture of food and saliva may run from the nose; this can be very distressing and if the choke does not spontaneously clear within 60 minutes then veterinary help should be sought. The vet may inject smooth muscle relaxants to help relieve spasms of the oesophagus, after which the choke should clear as the obstruction is allowed to move.

Horses that are prone to choke should be fed well dampened feeds which have been thoroughly mixed. Their speed of eating can be slowed down by putting a salt lick or several large stones in the manger. Diluting the concentrate feed with plenty of bulk in the form of chaff or soaked sugar beet pulp may be helpful. Some greedy horses which tend to choke on cubes should be fed a coarse mix instead. Dry coarse hay should be avoided and the teeth regularly checked for sharp edges and rasped when necessary.

Colic

Colic is not a disease but an abdominal pain (Fig. 13.1) which may be caused by a wide variety of disorders. The primary cause of this pain is distension of the stomach or intestines which may be due to an accu-

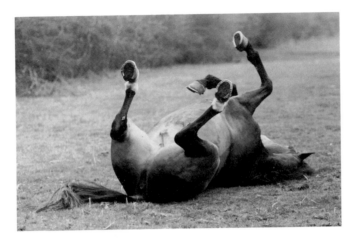

Fig. 13.1 Violent rolling can be a sign of colic.

mulation of gas, fluid or feed caused by a blockage or improper movement of the gut. Generally, the vet should be called as soon as colic is suspected; hay and feed should be removed and the horse left alone, unless it is so violent as to be in danger of injuring itself, in which case it should be walked and kept warm.

Spasmodic colic

Spasmodic colic is caused by spasm of the muscular wall of the intestine. There may be several reasons for this including: damage to the intestinal wall by migrating redworm larvae, a sudden change in diet, irregular feeding times, anxiety, tiredness or feeding and drinking too soon after fast work. Affected horses are usually moderately distressed. They usually pass few droppings. The condition may come and go quite quickly. If it persists, treatment with a relaxant drug usually relieves the problem rapidly.

Impactive colic

Impactive colic is caused by impaction of food material in the large intestine. This often occurs at the pelvic flexure where the intestine narrows near the pelvis to turn back towards the chest. It may occur because the horse has eaten its bedding or when it is brought in from grass, going onto a hay ration. Affected horses are not usually in a great deal of pain and tend to look dull and off-colour, getting up and down in an uncomfortable manner and rolling more than usual. The vet will insert a hand into the horse's rectum to try to feel where the blockage is; he or she may give the horse pain killers and also large amounts of liquid paraffin, or similar agent, via a stomach tube to stimulate gut movement.

Distension (tympanic) colic

Distension colic is caused by a buildup of gas in the gut and is usually very painful. Horses will sweat and roll violently, often hurting themselves in the process. Gas buildup may occur in front of an impaction and may be due to a twist in the gut or be caused by fermentation of food in the stomach or small intestine.

Twisted gut

Twisted gut, also known as intestinal catastrophe, is the most dramatic and serious form of colic. The intestines become twisted, telescoped into themselves or rotated about the mesentary, all of which obstruct the blood supply. Horses become uncontrollably violent in their agony and immediate veterinary attention is vital if the horse is to survive, as abdominal surgery is necessary.

Predisposing factors

Most colics are due to a management problem. Knowing the type of situation which may lead to a colic should help you avoid the situation occurring in the first place. Predisposing factors include:

- Sudden access to large quantities of rich feed, e.g. grass clippings, cereals, fallen apples, lush grass
- A changed routine, new stable or new surroundings
- Irregular work and changes in feeding routine
- Working on a full stomach
- Exhaustion
- Feeding and/or watering too soon after fast work
- Mouldy feed
- A sudden change of diet
- Sharp teeth
- Greedy feeders.

Prevention

As with most problems, good stable management and correct feeding are the answer to preventing colic.

- Feed each horse as an individual, noting its idiosyncrasies.
- Feed concentrates little and often, keeping to regular feeding times – even at weekends.
- Make changes to the diet gradually; do not increase concentrates by more than 0.5 kg (1.1 lb) a day when building up a ration.
- Have a planned, regular exercise programme.
- Feed good quality feed and store it away from vermin.
- Keep to your routine, even when away from home.
- Do not work the horse for at least 1 hour after feeding.
- Cool the horse thoroughly after strenuous work before allowing it to drink and eat large amounts.
- Have the teeth checked and rasped regularly.
- Stop horses bolting their feed by adding chaff or putting a salt lick or large stones in the manger.
- Keep to a regular, effective worming programme.

Diarrhoea

Diarrhoea or scouring can vary from being mild to life-threatening. Loose droppings can be due to several factors:

- Feeding and digestive problems
- A sudden change of diet, for example being turned out to grass
- Worms
- Excitement or nervousness
- Antibiotic treatments
- Bowel infection
- Poisoning.

Diarrhoea due to excitement should be fairly short term, with the droppings returning to the normal consistency once the horse has settled. Any prolonged scouring needs to be investigated by the vet. If the horse has a temperature the vet should be called immediately. Scouring in foals should always be treated seriously as they can quickly dehydrate and become very ill.

Feeding-related causes of diarrhoea include:

- Lush grass – horses used to a hay and concentrate ration that are turned out to grass often have cowpat-like droppings due to the high water content of the grass and the sudden change of diet. Once the horse's digestive system has accustomed itself to the grass the droppings should return to normal.
- Lack of fibre – horses receiving less than 50% fibre in the ration may have loose droppings. This is partly due to the lack of fibre in the diet and partly due to changes in the micro-organisms in the gut, leading to digestive disturbances.
- Too much water – bored horses may drink too much water.
- Poisonous plants.
- Sudden feed changes – loose droppings result from the upset to the micro-organisms of the gut and digestive disturbance. All feed changes must be made gradually.

Some horses have permanently loose droppings which appears to be related to a food allergy, a reaction to concentrated diets or the stress of work. These horses seem bright and alert but fail to hold their condition. They should be given a simple ration with added probiotics. Herbal mixtures designed to soothe the gut may prove helpful.

Azoturia

Azoturia is also known as 'tying-up', setfast, exertional rhabdomyolysis or 'Monday morning' disease. It is a condition where the muscles of the loins and hindquarters seize up, leading to stiffness and pain. Traditionally the problem arises soon after the onset of exercise, particularly in fit horses, maintained on a full ration, the day after a rest day. The signs vary from slight hind leg stiffness to severe pain and total reluctance to move. However, horses have been known to develop symptoms at grass, in the 10-minute box of a three-day event or during walking exercise. Some horses are prone to recurrent attacks and highly strung horses, especially mares, are susceptible.

Whatever the cause, the result is muscle damage, releasing muscle enzymes into the bloodstream; these enzymes – creatine phosphokinase (CPK) and aspartate aminotransferace (AST) – are used to assess the severity of the attack, and the speed at which the levels in the blood fall is used to monitor the rate of recovery from an attack. Lactic acid is also released from the damaged muscle cells and continuing to work a mildly affected horse can make the condition much worse; it is vital to stop work immediately and get the horse back to its box with as little energy expenditure as possible.

Treatment involves reduction of pain and inflammation. The horse may need to be sedated and have fluid therapy and it is important to keep it warm. It should be given only hay and water plus any medicines prescribed by the vet. Vitamin E and selenium have been used, but there is little information to support this and opinion seems to suggest an electrolyte imbalance as being a key point.

Prevention is through careful stable management and attention to diet.

- Reduce the concentrates if the horse has a day off.
- Warm up and cool down the horse properly.
- Make any changes to the diet gradually.
- Make sure that the diet contains adequate calcium, phosphorus and salt (sodium chloride).
- Use electrolytes to replace the salts lost when the horse sweats.
- Feed good quality hay and a low energy, low protein feed, for example horse and pony cubes, to susceptible horses.
- Turn the horse out to grass as much as possible.

Laminitis

Laminitis is inflammation of the sensitive laminae of the foot. In the UK it tends to be associated with overfat ponies and horses kept at grass, especially in the spring when the grass is growing very rapidly. It is also associated with grain overload (excessive carbohydrate consumption) and with generalised toxaemia, for example severe diarrhoea. However, any overweight, underexercised horse on a high grain ration is susceptible.

Causes of laminitis include:

- Lush or fast growing grass or clover, for example after rain during a dry summer
- Eating large amounts of food
- Toxaemia due to retained afterbirth, colic or diarrhoea

- Concussion from working on hard ground
- Irregular or incorrect hoof trimming
- Stress
- Allergy to drugs, e.g. corticosteroids
- Pituitary gland tumours in old ponies.

Any of the feet can be affected, but most commonly the forefeet. At first the horse may only take uneven steps when ridden, but if the warning signs are ignored it will soon be very reluctant to move, standing with its hind legs well under the body, and rocking back on the heels of the forefeet to take some weight off the toes. The extreme pain occurs because the blood supply to the foot is disturbed so that the sensitive laminae are starved of blood and the cells are damaged and die, causing inflammation and pain. In severe cases the pedal bone within the foot rotates and may even be forced through the sole of the hoof.

Treatment should eliminate the cause and alleviate the pain. Prompt treatment can make a significant difference to how well the horse recovers from laminitis. The vet may do several things:

- Give a laxative, such as liquid paraffin, via a stomach tube
- Give antibiotics in case of infection
- Give anti-inflammatory drugs
- Give pain killers
- Give a tranquilliser to calm an anxious horse and to bring down blood pressure
- Give a vasodilator to encourage the blood flow through the foot.

If the pedal bone is stable, walking on soft ground is important to encourage blood flow, but this should be limited to 10 minutes every 2 hours. The horse must not be walked if the pedal bone is rotating or exercise makes the feet more painful. The feet can be bathed in warm water to increase the blood supply to the foot, but this is unlikely to make much difference to the horse's recovery. The horse should be bedded on shavings or a similar bedding which supports the sole of the foot. Your veterinary surgeon will advise you.

Feeding the laminitic horse or pony

If the cause of the laminitis is overeating, the horse must be confined to the stable or a small starvation paddock, bare of grass. The diet must be restricted to water and a small amount of hay. The horse must not be literally starved as this can result in hyperlipaemia, a high concentration of lipids in the blood caused by breakdown of body fat; the horse with hyperlipaemia will lose its appetite, be depressed, lose coordination and become weak.

Supplementary minerals and vitamins are important when the diet is severely restricted like this. The horse should be fed a full dose of a general purpose mineral and vitamin supplement given in a double handful of low sugar chaff. Once the horse is recovering it should be fed a maintenance ration based on good quality hay. The concentrate ration should be based on digestible fibre, perhaps including alfalfa chaff, unmolassed sugar beet pulp and high fibre horse and pony cubes. A suitable supplement, perhaps one that encourages hoof growth and horn quality, can also be included. It may also be useful to feed a probiotic to try to keep the conditions within the gut as stable as possible. High starch and high sugar feeds should be avoided. If more energy or condition is needed oil can be added to the ration.

The fat pony may benefit from having part of the hay ration replaced by straw. Straw acts as a filler to keep the pony happy, without providing too much energy. Many owners are so anxious about their pony's laminitis re-occurring that they keep the pony too thin. There is no reason why the recovered laminitic should not be fed and worked as any other pony. However, the owner must be very vigilant about sudden changes to the ration or the grazing. It is these changes that will spark off another attack.

Any horse that has had laminitis is prone to further attacks and should be managed accordingly; access to pasture must be limited and bodyweight strictly controlled. Great care must be taken to be aware of any changes in the grass growth, for example if it rains after a dry spell in the summer the horse should be stabled and only allowed to graze for a short time every day.

Lymphangitis

The lymphatic system is a network of fine tubes which collect excess fluid from all parts of the body and return it to the bloodstream; the return of lymph is aided by muscle massage. Too little exercise and excess feeding leads to waterlogging in the tissues and the legs become filled with lymph fluid. This filling should go down after exercise.

Lymphangitis occurs when the walls of the blood and lymph vessels are damaged by toxins, so that water passes into the tissue spaces very quickly. The damage may be due to an allergic reaction to a feed or a drug, or may be a direct result of a viral or bacterial infection. A scab is often found on the lower part of the affected leg. Diets high in protein may aggravate the swellings due to the nutritional element adding to the drainage problem.

Lymphangitis usually occurs in the hind limb and may lead to a permanently enlarged limb. Treatment aims to combat infection and relieve pain so that controlled exercise can be given. The amount and type of feed must be looked at and changed if necessary. Generally, horse and pony cubes, mashes and hay are recommended. Rich grass should be avoided.

Allergies (urticaria, hives, nettlerash)

The natural response of the skin to allergic reactions may be the sudden appearance of variable sized lumps; a fairly common allergic reaction is to animal proteins in concentrate feeds and fresh grass proteins. The horse develops many small, firm bumps on the body which may be very itchy and the horse may go off its feed. This reaction is also known as urticaria, hives or nettlerash. The horse should have the concentrate part of the diet reduced right down, feeding bran mashes with Epsom salts and hay until the condition has resolved. Once the horse has recovered it is wise to avoid barley and high performance concentrates until the cause of the problem has been identified.

Dehydration

Dehydration is the excessive loss of water from the body tissues and may follow prolonged sweating in working horses or severe diarrhoea in horses suffering from salmonella infection or redworm infection. The adult horse's body is approximately 65–75% water and the foal's is 75–80% water and this is vital for life; any excess loss of water is bound to have serious consequences. The horse not only loses water but also important electrolytes, including sodium, potassium and sodium chloride. These electrolytes are involved in maintaining the correct volume and water content of the body cells; the horse must keep the cellular levels of these minerals within strict limits if it is to stay healthy. Any loss of fluids and electrolytes must be made good rapidly, especially in young stock, as dehydration can kill surprisingly rapidly. After work, dehydrated horses should be given about 4.5 l (1 gallon) water every 15 minutes, containing 30 g (1 oz) electrolytes.

If the horse will not drink, electrolyte replacement may be intravenous or via a stomach tube, using an electrolyte solution containing sodium chloride (common salt), glucose, lactate, potassium, calcium and magnesium; your veterinary surgeon will advise you. If the dehydration is mild then electrolytes in the water or feed for several days may be adequate.

Horses should be allowed to drink often during long periods of work. If the weather is very hot then 2 minutes' drinking every 2 hours is indicated; this way the horse will take water little and often. Large amounts of water may be harmful and the working horse is only able to utilize small drinks efficiently.

Chapter 14
Feeding and Temperament

At the first sign of a buck or an unnecessary spook most people blame the feed, prompting the feed manufacturers to produce 'cool' mixes and 'non-heating' cubes. We all know of overexuberant horses and their owners' search for a feed that will calm them down. Is the relationship between feeding and temperament that simple? Does what and how you feed really affect the way your horse behaves?

The horse in its natural state

Chapter 1 describes how the horse evolved and how the environment in which we keep horses is vastly different from that which really suits them. We have taken the modern horse and enclosed it in paddocks and stables, dramatically changing its life style and feeding habits. Its feeding time has been greatly reduced and we have introduced cereals and protein concentrates. No wonder horses are prone to temperament problems, stable 'vices', colic and other problems associated with feeding. Think of what we do to our horses' digestive systems: we give them additives, supplements and large quantities of highly processed concentrate feeds at times that fit in with our schedule. Add to this medications, wormers, antibiotics and pain killers and you can see that their diet is hugely different from their natural grazing habit.

The 'heating' effect of feed

There is no doubt that some horse react dramatically to small changes in their diet while others seem to tolerate large amounts of 'heating' feeds with no ill effects. There are three main reasons for the temperament changes associated with the way horses and ponies are fed:

- Too much energy
- Indigestion
- Nutrient imbalances.

Too much energy

Many naughty or overexuberant horses are simply getting too much food and not enough work. This situation is made worse by long hours spent standing in the stable with nothing to occupy their minds. Very often reducing the hard feed, increasing the hay ration and turning the horse out as much as possible can work wonders. Most horse owners enjoy mixing up feeds for their horses and persuading owners to feed less is often tricky. Hence, most of the 'non-heating' mixes and cubes are low energy, low protein and high fibre feeds which do not over-supply energy. Problems can arise here with Thoroughbreds which tend to have excitable temperaments and are often poor-doers and yet need plenty of food to keep condition, especially during the winter. These horses may benefit from additions to the diet such as oil, yeasts and probiotics.

Indigestion

The horse's digestive system was designed to extract nourishment from the fibre contained in grass by slow microbial fermentation in the hind gut. As we demand more work of the horse we have traditionally added cereal-based feeds to the ration. The energy in cereals is in the form of starches and sugars which are digested in the small intestine. Food only stays in the small intestine about 45 minutes and this does not always allow enough time for the complex starch molecules to be digested. Any starch passing through into the large intestine is rapidly fermented by the intestinal micro-organisms to produce lactic acid. There is an increase in the acidity of the gut (acidosis) which may lead to discomfort and a serious disturbance in the balance of fibre-digesting bacteria. Feeding processed cereals improves the rate of digestion in the small intestine, reduces hind gut fermentation and keeps the horse's metabolism more stable. Figure 14.1 shows the difference in the way the horse digests cereal and its natural feed, fibrous grass.

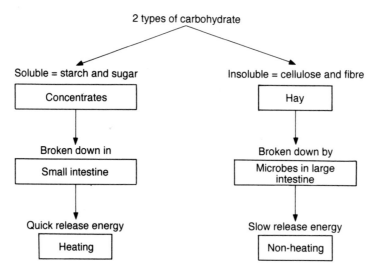

Fig. 14.1   Carbohydrate digestion.

Nutrient imbalances

Some minerals and vitamins play an important role in the function of the horse's nervous system and an imbalance of these substances appears to affect the way the horse behaves. Substances such as potassium, magnesium, chromium, amino acids and B vitamins are sometimes used in additives to maintain calmness and reduce anxiety.

Guidelines for feeding the temperamental horse

- Do not feed too much.
- Follow the 'rules of good feeding' (see Chapter 2).
- Feed as few concentrates and as much hay as possible, taking into consideration the horse's work level and condition.
- Feed high fibre, low starch, concentrate feeds.
- Instead of feeding more concentrates to horses that need more condition, try adding a yeast culture.
- Use probiotics in times of stress.
- Seek advice if a temperament problem continues: the horse could be in pain and trying to tell you something.

What to feed

Except for high performance horses, the lower the starch in the diet and the higher the fibre the happier the horse will be. So how can we provide the energy the horse needs for work?

Fat

The first things the weight watcher has to cut out are high fat foods – cream, butter, cheese and chocolate. Fat is a very concentrated source of energy, containing nearly two-and-a-half times as much energy as starch. Fats and oils are efficiently digested in the small intestine, so we can add extra 'non-heating' energy to the horse's ration by including oil.

Fibre

Digestible fibre can provide a natural 'non-heating' energy source for working horses. Fibre sources include cereal and oilseed meals, grass, alfalfa, and sugar beet. When choosing a feed, look at the fibre level as well as the energy and protein levels. Some horse and pony cubes are essentially cereal-free, providing energy from fibre sources such as grassmeal, wheatfeed and oatfeed. Wheatfeed and oatfeed are the outer fibrous covering of the cereal grain. It is now possible to buy high fibre competition feeds that still have suitable levels of energy and protein. Due to the nature of the manufacturing process, cubes tend to have a higher fibre level than the equivalent mix, a useful point to remember when feeding the temperamental horse.

Processed feed

For years we have used boiled barley to put condition on lean horses; cooking it makes it more 'fattening'. Cooking processes such as steam flaking, extrusion and micronisation result in the unravelling of the complex starch molecule into a more easily digestible form. As more of the starch can then be broken down and absorbed in the small intestine there is less likely to be an excess of starch spilling over into the large intestine, helping to avoid the equine equivalent of indigestion. All these processes are used to treat ingredients of coarse mixes, increasing digestibility and inactivating some toxic factors.

Yeasts

Some feeds now contain yeast cultures which improve fibre digestion by stimulating the bacteria in the large intestine. They are also thought to help stabilise the conditions in the gut, counteracting the effects of a high starch diet.

Enzymes

Some supplements make use of enzymes. These help break down the food into substances small enough to be absorbed across the gut wall. Enzymes make the feed more digestible, allowing the horse owner to feed fewer concentrates or for the horse to put on condition.

Absorbent, demulcent clays

Some digestive aids consist of very fine clays. The swelling action of these clays is said to slow down the rate of passage of food, allowing more efficient digestion. It is also claimed that they have the ability to absorb acid, thus maintaining a healthy gut environment. Removing the acid from the gut calms horses down by removing the discomfort associated with chronic digestive upset.

Probiotics

The horse's gut is populated by bacteria which are essential for the proper digestion of fibre and the health of the horse. These bacteria are susceptible to changes in the horse's gut caused by changes in feeding, strenuous exercise, travelling, irregular feeding and changes in surroundings – in other words, stress. Probiotics are live, microbial feed supplements that help the normal bacteria and other naturally occurring gut micro-organisms to maintain a stable, healthy environment. Probiotics can be live cultures of bacteria or a non-viable product of bacterial fermentation. Using probiotics is by no means a new idea – they are what makes 'live' yoghurt.

Probiotics are thought to reduce the effects of stress on the gut micro-organisms in several ways:

- By changing the micro-organisms in the gut and reducing the incidence of disease-causing *E. coli*
- By stimulating immunity to other bacteria
- By colonising the digestive tract
- By producing stimulating substances
- By reducing toxic substances.

Probiotics are used in agriculture as a natural alternative to hormone implants and infeed antibiotics. They are produced from known beneficial bacteria, cultured under strict quality control in the laboratory, preserved to maintain viability and formulated for oral administration. They have been shown to control scouring and improve growth in foals.

Most probiotics fed to horses are a blend of different strains of bacteria. They are protected to survive the acidity of the stomach so that they pass into the intestine, where they colonise. They are presented as pastes to be administered orally or as a compound to be added to the feed. Probiotics help restore the natural balance of the gut microflora so that the horse can quickly return to its normal nutrition, growth and health status.

Correcting nutrient imbalances

If, despite feeding small amounts of high fibre feed, your horse still has an unreliable or excitable temperament, it may be due to a nutrient imbalance.

Herbs

Herbs have long played an important role in medicine in all cultures, worldwide and it is assumed that they correct a nutrient imbalance. The principle of herbal treatments is that the whole body is affected; herbs restore balance and harmony to the body's systems, including the nervous system. The calming effects of certain herbs have been well documented. Valerian, chamomile and hops are said to encourage relaxation of the nervous system and muscles. The effects of feeding herbs are cumulative and build up slowly so they must be given adequate time to work. Specialist equine herbalists will make you up a herbal mix to suit your horse depending on its individual problems.

Potassium and magnesium

Stabled performance horses being fed restricted amounts of hay and subjected to hard work resulting in sweating may experience a shortage of potassium and magnesium. Sudden stress or dietary changes, such as a flush of spring grass, can increase the horse's need for magnesium. Magnesium loss has been associated with temperament problems and misbehaviour.

Amino acids and B vitamins

The amino acid L-tryptophan and vitamin B_1 (thiamine) can be added to the diet to maintain calmness and relaxation.

Chapter 15
Stud Stock and Youngstock

The Thoroughbred industry has spent much time and money investigating the nutritional requirements and feeding management of breeding horses. Many large stud farms employ a nutritionist to analyse the nutritional value of their grazing, hay and concentrate feed. This allows them to design balanced rations for stallions, pregnant and lactating brood mares and for youngsters at all stages of growth. Some of the feed companies that specialise in making compound feeds for stud stock offer free nutritional help and advice; this may include a visit from their nutritionist and grassland and forage analysis. The main problems arise with the non-professional horse breeder who is perhaps breeding a foal from a favourite mare or has bought a foal to grow on. There is little in books to tell you how to feed native pony youngsters or fat, cob mares.

The brood mare

Getting the mare in foal

The mare's oestrous cycle is governed by daylight and mares will come into season every 21 days from the onset of spring. Pregnancy lasts for 11 months so most foals are born naturally in early summer. Mares that are thin or are losing condition are more difficult to get in foal than mares in good condition (Fig. 15.1) so it is important to ensure that the mare looks well before going to stud. For the mare in good condition, a maintenance ration of good quality hay until Christmas should be adequate. If you want an early foal she should be stabled at night at around Christmas, rugged, given 16 hours of light a day and fed a concentrate feed once or twice a day. The idea is to persuade the mare's body systems that spring is on the way, and this starts her oestrous cycle earlier in the year than normal. If you are happy to have

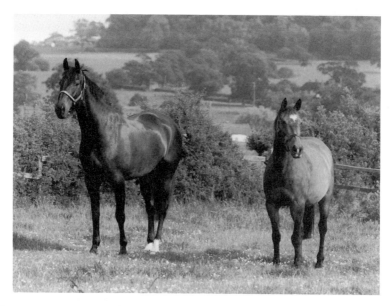

Fig. 15.1   Mares in good condition.

a later foal, the mare is a good-doer and your fields are not too wet she may live out all winter.

Thoroughbred horses and mares that tend to lose condition during the winter may need to be stabled at night and fed concentrates and hay to appetite. The amount of concentrates will depend on the size and type of horse as well as the weather conditions, the access to grass and the quality of the hay. Cold, wet weather will increase the mare's maintenance requirements and she will need more concentrate feed. The guidelines for feeding horses in winter should be used. Like all other horses, brood mares should follow an effective worming programme, have their teeth rasped regularly and have their feet trimmed when necessary.

Overweight mares which are being fed a low energy diet to reduce their weight have been shown to be more difficult to get in foal than fat mares which are fed to maintain their weight. This means that very fat mares should be dieted well before going to stud and then maintained at a constant bodyweight for 4–6 weeks immediately before going away to stud. In terms of condition score, the ideal is about 3, with the mare in fit but not fat condition. If the mare is very fit she should be 'let down' for 4–6 weeks before being sent to stud. If she is on the lean side she should be fed to gain condition.

Early pregnancy

The in-foal mare should be kept as naturally as possible so that she stays relaxed, happy and healthy. Overfeeding is detrimental to the mare's health and the subsequent condition of the newborn foal. During the first 8 months of pregnancy the fetus grows very little and, unless the mare has a foal at foot or is working, she can be fed for maintenance. In other words, she is fed to maintain her bodyweight in fit but not fat or thin condition; her ribs should not be visible, but they should be easily detected on touch, with no thick layer of fat disguising them. This will make foaling easier and enhance her chances of getting in foal again. Many owners tend to overfeed their mares during pregnancy; feeding the mare more will not result in a larger, stronger foal. In practical terms this means that from the time she is tested in-foal until October, good quality pasture should satisfy all her nutrient requirements. In dry summers, it may be necessary to feed hay or horse and pony cubes to make up for the lack of grass.

If the mare is overweight she can be put on a 'diet' after she has been in foal for 3 months. However, trying to get her to lose weight by underfeeding energy during the very early stages of pregnancy may result in the mare losing the foal. The fat mare should have any concentrate feed gradually removed from the diet, her access to grazing restricted and, if possible, she should be ridden as well. If ridden exercise is not possible she could be put on a horse walker for 20–30 minutes two or three times a week. The obese mare must not be starved or fed poor quality hay which is likely to be deficient in protein and vitamins and minerals.

Late pregnancy: the last 3 months

The growing fetus makes very few demands on the mare during the first 8 months of pregnancy. Although a tremendous amount of development is taking place, the fetus is not actually growing fast enough to make any appreciable demands on the mare. During the last 3 months of pregnancy the fetus starts to grow rapidly and the mare's nutrient requirements increase. At the same time, the fetus begins to occupy a greater proportion of the mare's abdomen, there is less room for her gut and consequently her appetite for bulk feed may fall; this must be made up by feeding a greater proportion of concentrate feed. As a guideline, the level of concentrate feed and hay should be increased by an average of 10% per month for the last 3 months before foaling.

The mare's nutrient requirements increase so that the developing foal's body tissue can be laid down; this requires both energy and protein. The pregnant mare requires about 12% protein in her diet overall. Even good quality hay will only have a protein content of about 10%; this means that every kilogram of hay fed leads to a shortfall of protein of 2%. In order to overcome this deficiency the mare's concentrate feed should have a protein content of about 16%. This means feeding a compound cube or mix specially formulated for breeding animals or adding soyabean meal to a cereal-based ration. In order to raise sufficiently the protein level of an oat-based ration, 0.5 kg (1.1 lb) soyabean meal should be fed for every 4 kg (8.8 lb) oats.

In winter, the mare may need to come in at night, although there are no hard and fast rules; a part-bred mare may be happier outside. A mare does not have to be stabled just because she is in foal. Now is the time to start introducing a concentrate feed unless, as with some native breeds, she is overweight. The mare's feed should be gradually increased so that she maintains her condition; a 16.2-hh (164-cm) Thoroughbred mare may need as much as 6.3–7.3 kg (14–16 lb) concentrate feed per day. It is equally important not to overfeed brood mares; it is a fallacy that only fat ponies are susceptible to laminitis – overfed, barren and pregnant mares are equally at risk.

There is conflicting evidence concerning the effects of overfeeding and underfeeding in the last 3 months of pregnancy. Generally, the fat mare should maintain, not lose, weight and the thin mare should gain weight. Any imposed weight loss in obese, pregnant mares should take place between the second and eighth month of pregnancy, and pre-ferably before they are covered (sent to stud).

During late pregnancy the mare needs higher levels of calcium and phosphorus for bone development in the unborn foal; this is particu-larly true for the older mare. Mares being fed a cereal-based diet should be given 42 g (2 tablespoons) dicalcium phosphate every day. At foaling, the calcium requirement increases by 50% as the mare pro-duces milk for the foal. If you live in an area known to be copper-deficient it is wise to consult a vet or nutritionist about introducing a copper supplement into the ration. The mare has a greater requirement for vitamin A during late pregnancy and will also need adequate levels of vitamin D to ensure proper use of the calcium in the diet; these can be supplied by feeding cod liver oil.

Table 15.1 shows a sample ration. As always, any ration cited is only a guide; all horses are individuals and must be treated as such. The concentrate may be in the form of a high protein (15%) stud cube.

Table 15.1 Sample ration for a 16-hh (162-cm), 500-kg (1100-lb), lightweight mare in the last 3 months of pregnancy.

Digestible energy	10.5 MJ DE/kg of diet
Crude protein	11%
Ratio of medium quality hay to concentrates	65:35
Calcium	0.5%
Phosphorus	0.35%
Ratio of calcium to phosphorus	1.5:1
Hay of 8 MJ DE/kg	8 kg (18 lb)
Concentrate of 12 MJ DE/kg	3–4 kg (6–9 lb)

Foaling

Some mares may naturally go off their feed as foaling approaches. Do not panic; lower her concentrate ration and let her eat as much good quality hay as she wants. In later foaling mares, the flush of spring grass will occur at about this time and may help reduce the problem of meconium (the foal's first droppings) retention. In the 24 hours before foaling, the mare should be fed good quality hay and low energy concentrates, e.g. horse and pony cubes with chaff, bran or sugar beet pulp. It is likely that the mare will go off her feed anyway. The first feed after foaling may usefully be a bran mash, as this is appetising and easy to eat, though bran is controversial as it upsets the calcium to phosphorus ratio of the ration. Bran mashes should always be supplemented with limestone flour or dicalcium phosphate. The now lactating mare will subsequently go onto a higher plane of nutrition.

Lactation

Many owners overfeed young, growing horses and pregnant mares, but underfeed lactating mares. Mares should be fed to maintain their good condition. Once a mare foals and starts to produce milk to feed her foal she needs more energy, protein, calcium, vitamin A and other minerals and vitamins. Her requirement for energy increases by up to 70% and for protein by up to 60% compared with late pregnancy. In other words, her energy and protein requirements are comparable with a horse in very hard work. The way a mare is fed after foaling will affect how quickly she comes back into season and thus how quickly she can be put back in foal. Mares that lose weight after foaling may take an extra 30 days to come back into season, while thin, stressed mares may take as long as 80 days. Obese mares can afford to lose some weight slowly after foaling without affecting milk production and fertility.

The body condition of mares with foals at foot (Fig. 15.2) should be regularly monitored and hay or extra concentrates given if they show any signs of losing condition. This is particularly important during dry summers when there may be a shortage of grazing. It is vital that mares have access to adequate water; during peak lactation they can produce 15–20 1 (3.5–4.5 gallons) milk and obviously need to drink large amounts to produce this milk. Lack of water will soon reduce milk production.

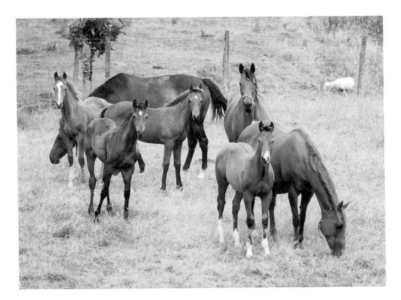

Fig. 15.2   Mares with foals at foot.

If mares foal when nature intended, in other words to coincide with abundant spring grass, this should meet all her requirements for energy, protein, calcium and phosphorus. Early foaling mares being fed low protein, grass hay and with limited access to grass will need a stud diet with 16–17% crude protein. The mare should not be overfed roughage as this may limit her capacity for concentrate; the hay to concentrate ratio will need to be higher than for pregnancy in order to meet the higher protein requirement.

A cereal mix can replace the high protein (15%) stud cube fed in the last 3 months of pregnancy, but it must be supplemented with soyabean meal or another protein concentrate. A 550-kg (1100-lb) mare on a grass hay and oat/barley diet would need 1.75 kg (3.8 lb) soyabean meal a day to bring the protein level of the ration up to 12.5%. It is very important to add salt and limestone/dicalcium phosphate to this cereal-based ration as well as a mineral and vitamin mix. As the foal grows it eats more and more grass and the mare's milk production gradually declines, so after about 3 months the concentrate feed can be gradually reduced, so that when the foal is weaned the mare is on a hay/grass-only diet. Table 15.2 shows a sample ration. Salt, dicalcium phosphate and cod liver oil may also be fed.

The stallion

Out of the breeding season the stallion in good condition (Fig. 15.3) should maintain his condition on good quality hay and horse and pony cubes. This plane of nutrition should be gradually increased after Christmas, as exercise is introduced to fitten him for the covering season. During the covering season, stallions may become difficult to feed, refusing to eat and losing condition. They should be fed a stud cube or equivalent concentrate mix and good quality hay at the rate of 3–4 kg (6–9 lb) for a 16.2-hh (164-cm), Thoroughbred stallion of 500 kg (1100 lb). Generally, the stallion should be fed as if he is doing moderately hard work, with good quality palatable feed and a general mineral and vitamin supplement. While a deficiency of vitamin E has been implicated in fertility problems, feeding extra vitamin E does not guarantee extra fertility! Pony stallions should not be allowed to become too fat. The basis of the diet should be hay which is topped by 1 or 2 hours' grazing every day. If

Table 15.2 Sample ration for a 16-hh (162-cm), 500-kg (1100-lb), lightweight, lactating mare.

Early lactation (first 3 months)	
Digestible energy	12 MJ DE/kg of diet
Crude protein	12.5%
Ratio of hay to concentrates	60:40
Calcium	0.5%
Phosphorus	0.35%
Ratio of calcium to phosphorus	1.5:1
Hay of 8 MJ DE/kg	6–7 kg (13–15 lb) and/or grass
Concentrate of 12 MJ DE/kg	4–5.5 kg (9–12 lb)
Second 3 months of lactation	
Digestible energy	11 MJ DE/kg diet
Crude protein	11%
Ratio of hay to concentrates	70:30
Calcium	0.45%
Phosphorus	0.3%
Ratio of calcium to phosphorus	1.5:1
Hay of 8 MJ DE/kg	8–9 kg (18–20 lb) and/or grass
Concentrate of 12 MJ DE/kg	3–4 kg (6–9 lb)

the stallion is too fat he should not be starved but put on a balanced weight reduction diet and worked under saddle or on the lunge every day.

Guide to feeding mares and stallions (Table 15.3)

Remember that all horses are individuals and their feed requirements will depend on

- When the mare is due to foal
- The quantity of grazing
- The quality of grazing
- Breed
- Type.

Fat horses should be fed less than the guidelines and a broad-spectrum mineral supplement added to the diet.

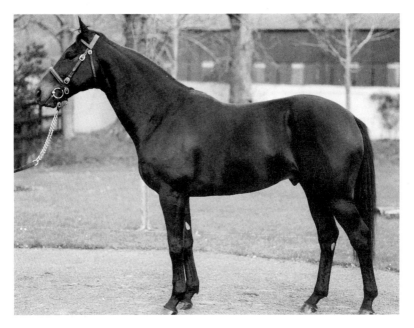

Fig. 15.3 A stallion.

Youngstock

Rapidly growing young horses are prone to a number of conditions related to development and feeding, known as developmental ortho-paedic diseases. These problems can be sparked off by overfeeding, underfeeding, imbalanced diets and inconsistent feeding practices. It is crucial that the horse grows at an optimum rate which is controlled by a combination of balanced nutrition, well managed feeding regimes and suitable exercise.

Newly born foals

The newborn foal must suckle sufficient colostrum from its mother within 8–12 hours of being born. Colostrum is the mare's first milk and it contains high levels of antibodies to help protect the foal from disease during the first few weeks of life. Foals that do not get enough colostrum tend to be weak and more susceptible to infectious disease. If you are not sure that a foal has drunk enough colostrum, consult your vet.

Table 15.3   Feeding mares and stallions.

	In foal mares: last 3 months of pregnancy	Lactating mares: foaling to 3 months	Mares: 4 months to weaning	Stallions: during the stud season
Welsh Section A (250 kg/550 lb)	1.25–2 kg 3–4 lb	2–2.5 kg 4–5.5 lb	1.25–2 kg 3–4 lb	1.25–2 kg 3–4 lb
Connemara (400 kg/900 lb)	2–3 kg 4–6.5 lb	3–4 kg 6.5–9 lb	2–3 kg 4–6.5 lb	2–3 kg 4–6.5 lb
Thoroughbred (550 kg/1210 lb)	2.75–4 kg 6–9 lb	4–5.5 kg 9–12 lb	2.75–4 kg 6–9 lb	2.75–4 kg 6–9 lb
Warmblood (650 kg/1430 lb)	3.25–5 kg 7–11 lb	5–6.5 kg 11–14 lb	3.25–5 kg 7–11 lb	3.25–5 kg 7–11 lb

Once the foal is up on its feet it will suckle (Fig. 15.4) about four times every hour, day and night, for the first week of its life. It will probably take very short drinks of perhaps no more than a minute. After the first week, foals suckle less often but tend to take longer drinks. Watch out for a foal that suckles very aggressively or frequently; it may be that the mare is short of milk and that the foal is hungry.

Most foals will start to nibble grass or to taste their mother's feed by the time they are a week old. These eating experiments contribute little to their overall nutrition. After about 2 or 3 weeks, foals will graze close to their mother. Providing that the mare is properly fed and has adequate milk, milk alone should supply all the foal's nutritional requirements. However, after about 3 months, the mare's milk yield starts to decline and the foal becomes more dependent on grass as a supply of nutrients. If you are short of grass the foal may need supplementary feeding. It is best to use a concentrate feed specially formulated as a 'creep' feed for foals. Correctly fed, these are designed to maintain an optimum rather than maximum rate of growth. Studies have shown that foals with even and steady growth rates before and after weaning are less likely to suffer from growth-related problems. Mangers specially designed for feeding mares and foals have an area for the foal creep feed which is too small for the mare to insert her muzzle. The young foal will need 0.5–1 kg (1.1–2.2 lb) creep feed per 100 kg (220 lb) bodyweight; this is 0.5–1.5 kg (1.1–3.3 lb) per day for

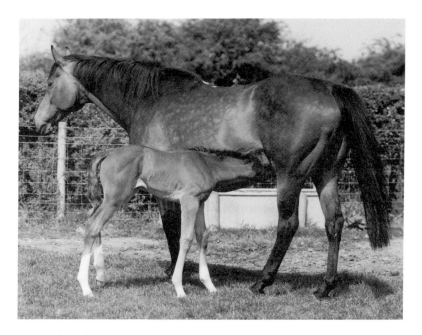

Fig. 15.4   A new foal suckling.

a foal which will make 16 hh (162 cm) at maturity. A rule of thumb is to feed 450 g (1 lb) creep feed per day for every month of age. Thus, a 4-month-old foal should receive 1.8 kg (4 lb) creep feed per day. Native breeds are unlikely to need creep feeding.

Weanlings (Fig. 15.5)

Most foals are weaned at about 6 months of age, and the next 6 months is one of the most critical growth periods. The young horse needs a steady growth rate and balanced nutrition. It is better for a foal to grow more slowly for longer than it is to grow very rapidly. This means that a young horse should not be overfed; many people like to keep their youngsters in lean but healthy condition, with a moderate condition score so that the ribs can be felt on pressure and the horse is not overfat. Youngsters that are being prepared for the show ring or for sale will need to carry more condition, but the ideal is to produce a well proportioned and athletic animal which is not carrying too much weight. This requires a careful combination of correct feeding and controlled exercise.

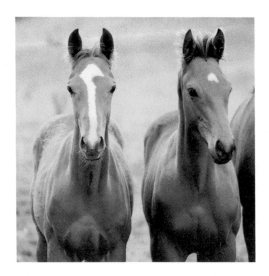

Fig. 15.5   Weanlings.

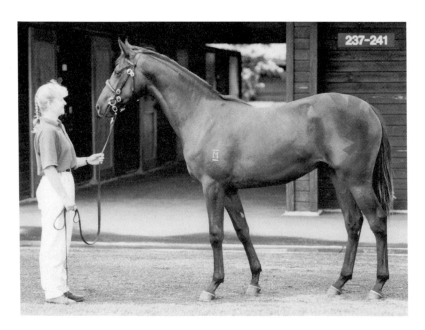

Fig. 15.6   Yearling prepared for sale.

Weaning is a traumatic time for foals and can result in a considerable setback in their growth if they have not been prepared for the change from a milk-based diet to a grass/hay/concentrate diet. Weaning should be well managed to reduce the stress on the young foal. Part of this management is to ensure that the foal has been supplemented with concentrate feed, either as a creep feed or by sharing its mother's feed. As a guideline, weanlings should be fed 1 kg (2.2 lb) per 100 kg (220 lb) body weight; this is 1.5–2 kg (3.3–4.4 lb) feed per day in a weanling expected to make 16 hh (162 cm) at maturity. The feed should contain about 15% crude protein and have an energy level around 12 MJ DE/kg. As the weanling grows, the feed must be increased accordingly, keeping an eye on the condition and limbs.

As the youngster gets older, its growth rate slows down and its requirement for protein falls so that a yearling (Fig. 15.6) needs about 0.75 kg (1.7 lb) feed per 100 kg (220 lb) bodyweight and the 2-year-old needs only 0.5 kg (1.1 lb).

Guide to feeding youngstock (Table 15.4)

Specially formulated compound mixes or pellets are probably the best choice of feed; making a ration at home that has the right levels of energy, protein, minerals and vitamins is likely to be difficult. Grain-based feeds and winter grass will be deficient in protein, calcium, copper, zinc and vitamins A and D. Like all horses, the amount of feed a youngster requires depends on:

- The quantity and quality of grazing
- Breed and type

Table 15.4 Feeding youngstock.

Age	Feed		Daily ration for a horse to make 16 hh (162 cm) and 500 kg (1100 lb) at maturity	
	(kg/100 kg bodyweight)	(lb/100 lb bodyweight)	(kg)	(lb)
0–6 months	0.5–1	1–2	0.5–1.5 (up to 2)	1–3
Weanling	1	2	1.5–2 (up to 4)	3–4.5
Yearling	0.75	1.5	2–3 (up to 5)	4.5–6.5
2-year old	0.5	1	1.5–2 (up to 4)	3–4.5

- Weather conditions
- Hay quality.

Overfat youngsters should be put on a maintenance diet of good quality hay, a reduced level of concentrates and broad-spectrum mineral and vitamin supplement. They should also be exercised in hand or on the lunge in such a way as to help them lose weight without putting too much strain on the limbs.

Growth-related disorders in young, growing horses can be avoided by:

- Providing a balanced ration
- Not overfeeding quantity
- Not oversupplying energy
- Aiming for steady growth rates
- Avoiding high growth rates, growth spurts and overdevelopment
- Ensuring adequate and regular exercise.

The orphan foal

The first thing when feeding the orphan foal is to ensure that it receives adequate colostrum. Then, if a foster mother cannot be found, the foal may have to be hand-reared. A feeding bottle can be made by fitting a clean, soft-drink bottle with a lamb teat. The foal should be taught to drink milk from a bucket as soon as possible; allowing the foal to lick milk off the fingers and then immersing the fingers in the bucket will encourage the foal to follow the finger and discover the milk. It must never be forced to put its head in the bucket.

If the foal is premature or lacks a normal suck reflex it must be fed through a stomach tube until it has learned to suckle. The foal's nostril should be greased and a soft rubber tube passed into the nostril, down the foal's throat. When the tube reaches the back of the throat the foal should swallow so that the tube passes down the gullet into the stomach, not into the lungs. The handler must listen to the end of the tube before putting any milk down the tube; if it is in the lungs a characteristic noise will be heard and the tube should be slowly withdrawn. A vet must show you how to use the stomach tube correctly. Milk at body temperature should then be slowly poured into a funnel attached to the tube.

A reputable mare's milk replacer, made up as directed, should be used; cow's milk is too rich, but goat's milk can be used. During the first 2 weeks, normal, healthy foals should be fed every 2 hours and during the second 2 weeks they should be fed every 4 hours. They should then be fed four times a day until weaning. Individual needs as to the amount and frequency of feeds will vary according to the foal's size, age and state of health, but initially foals should be fed about 300 ml (0.5 pt) at each feed. Each week the amount fed should be increased to the maximum that the foal will eat without scouring. Scouring without fever or any other signs of illness may indicate that the foal is being overfed and its diet should be adjusted accordingly.

The orphan foal should be introduced to solid feed as quickly as possible; this will encourage gut development and allow the foal to be weaned from the bucket earlier. Pellets containing milk or milk replacer pellets can be added to the bucket of milk replacer, which will encourage the foal to eat them. The pellets should contain at least 16–18% high quality protein, and have a high energy content and adequate levels of minerals and vitamins, particularly calcium and phosphorus. The hand-reared, orphan foal should be weaned from milk replacers as soon as possible; early weaning will save labour costs and allow the foal to lead a more normal life. The foal must look well and be eating adequate creep feed before the milk ration is gradually reduced and creep feeding continued for another 3 months.

General guidelines for feeding stud stock

- Feed good quality forage.
- If forage is not good quality make good the shortfall by feeding extra concentrates or alfalfa.
- Do not rely solely on pasture; its quality can vary dramatically depending on time of year, sward quality and soil nutrition. Compensate for pasture inadequancy with concentrates.
- Constantly check condition and growth rates to avoid poor conformation and developmental orthopaedic disease.
- Feed adequate calcium and phosphorus in the correct ratio and quantity.

- Only use one, good, general mineral, vitamin and amino acid supplement. Except in specific cases, the use of more than one supplement may imbalance the ration further, as they may not complement each other.

Appendix 1
Units

Conversions

1 kg = 2.205 lb	1 g = 1000 mg
1 lb = 0.454 kg	1000 g = 1 kg
1000 kg = 1 tonne	1000 ml = 1 litre
1 oz = 28.35 g	1 pint = 0.568 litres
1 g = 0.035 oz	4.544 litres = 1 gallon

Energy

This is given in the book as Digestible Energy (DE). Energy is measured in megajoules (MJ). DE is usually expressed in terms of how much energy there is in one kilogram of a food, so it is written as MJ/kg.

Grams per kilogram (g/kg)

This is a measure of the number of grams of one substance in a kilogram of another. An example would be the number of grams of a nutrient in one kilogram of food.

Percentages

This gives the amount of one thing expressed as part of 100 of another. If the amount of calcium in a food is 2%, it means that there are 2 g of calcium for every 100 g of the food. Percentages are another way of expressing a value as g/kg and both may be used in feed information.

International units

These are given in iu, and are used for vitamins A, D and E. The conversion is:

1 iu of vitamin A = 0.3 microgams
1 iu of vitamin D = 0.025 micrograms
1 iu of vitamin E = 1 milligram

Index